Handbook Guide to Kidney Transplant

Handbook Guide to Kidney Transplant

ASHRAF I. REYAD MB BCH

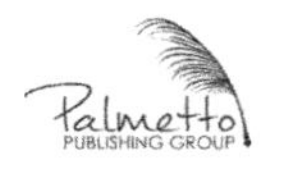

Palmetto Publishing Group
Charleston, SC

Handbook Guide to Kidney Transplant

This book is provided "as is" and the publisher and author disclaim any warranties, express or implied, including any warranties to accuracy, comprehensiveness, or currency of the content of this book.

This work is merely a reference tool and is not a substitute for individual patient assessment by healthcare professionals. It is the sole responsibility of healthcare professionals managing patients, and not the publisher, to assess each individual patient clinical considerations and management plans.

To the fullest extent of the law, neither the Publisher nor the Author assumes any liability for any injury and / or damage to persons or property , as a matter of products liability, negligence law or otherwise, or from any reference to or use by any person of this work. With the rapid evolving nature of research and best practice, readers are advised to check the most current information provided on medical diagnosis, indications, appropriate pharmaceutical selections and dosages and treatment options. These should be made and a verified through consulting a variety of sources. When prescribing medicine please see product information sheet accompanying each drug to verify indications, warnings, side effects, dosage, frequency and contraindications of use.

First Edition

Printed in the United States

Paperback ISBN: 978-1-64990-595-6
eBook ISBN: 978-1-64990-596-3

Dedication

To my beautiful wife, who has been the anonymous soldier in my journey, thank you for your patience and unwavering support. I am grateful for the opportunity that allowed me to have the time to write this book. To my mentors throughout the years, at the Royal College of Surgeons in Ireland, Sinai Hospital in Baltimore, and Johns Hopkins Hospital in Baltimore, who have guided me into becoming the physician I am today. To my patients, who are my teachers and motivation to be better.

Contents

Preface

The purpose of this book is to provide a compact and to-the-point update on kidney transplants. It is not a comprehensive book but rather a practical book that describes common practices and treatments and explores recent practices in kidney transplants. It covers the basic sciences of the subject and dives into landmark clinical trials. The aim of the book is to inspire best practice to take care of transplant patients.

Renal Anatomy

Kidneys: retroperitoneal organs.
The right kidney is slightly lower than the left (*due to the liver*).
The hilum of each kidney is at roughly L1 (*transpyloric plane*).
The upper pole is at T12, and the lower pole is at L2-L3.
They are surrounded by **Gerota's fascia**.
Posterior to kidneys: the diaphragm and costodiaphragmatic recess of the pleural cavity (*pneumothorax risk with inadvertent biopsy or injections*).
Anterior to the right kidney: ascending colon, hepatic flexure, duodenum.
Left kidney neighbors: the spleen, stomach, splenic flexure, descending colon.

Renal Arteries: arise from the aorta at L1. Considered end arteries, they *should be preserved as much as possible*, especially in the presence of accessory vessels.

Left: short.
Right: longer, but passes posterior to the inferior vena cava (IVC).
Accessory vessels: occur as kidneys ascend during fetal life. Most common: inferior pole arteries of the kidney, which usually supply ureters (*an important factor when assessing anatomy of donors*).

Renal Vein: drains into the IVC.

Right: short but no branching.
Left: drains adrenal and gonadal veins before crossing anterior to the aorta immediately below the superior mesenteric artery. (*Accessory veins are usually safe to be tied, especially if their diameter is less than 1/3 of the main renal vein.*)

Renal Pelvis / Ureter

Drainage: minor calyces → major calyces → renal pelvis → ureter.

The ureter:

1. Descends in line with the tip of the transverse process.
2. Crosses the pelvic brim anterior to the sacroiliac joint and common iliac artery bifurcation.
3. Enters medially and forward into the bladder at the ischial spine level.

(*Common sites of renal stone obstruction are the pelviureteric junction, pelvic brim crossing, and the bladder insertion.*)

Renal Embryology

Average total nephron count in humans: 750,000 (250,000–2,000,000,000).

Derived from the mesoderm (mesothelium/mesenchyme) and endoderm.

Combined with genital development → urogenital development in **three stages**.

The first two stages leave a rudimentary structure that sets a block for the next stage of development (von Baer's Law ancestral repetition of rudimentary structures).

A urogenital ridge arising from the intermediate mesoderm and on either side of the aorta forms the pronephros, mesonephros, and metanephros (from head to tail).

Stage 1:

Pronephros: Two draining ducts are derived from the mesenchymal tissue form close to the level of the heart and are the most cephalic end of the tube at week four. They are non-functional but lay the blueprint for future stages.

Stage 2:

The ducts become more elaborate and functional and continue caudally and drain into the cloaca. The midsection is referred to as the **mesonephros**. It develops a mesonephric duct (**Wolffian Duct**). The pronephros degenerates at this stage, and the mesonephros (first trimester kidney) takes over.

The mesonephros caudal portion that drains into the cloaca is called the **metanephros,** and this will develop into the kidney. The mesonephros degenerates, but its rudimentary tract, the Wolffian duct, and the paramesonephric tissue will develop into genital structures in both males and females.

Vascular buds from the kidney grow and invade the common iliac vessels. The kidney ascends from the pelvis toward the flanks during fetal development; in doing so new vascular buds invade more cranially, and the caudal branches regress. Sometimes, these *vessels don't regress* and result in supernumerary renal arteries, which in rare situations can *compress the ureters* and cause **hydronephrosis**.

Stage 3:

The metanephros will continue to develop tubules and ducts forming a ureteric bud that proliferates into the surrounding metanephric mesenchyme called the **metanephric blastema**. The ureteric bud proliferates due to growth factors from the blastema and develops everything from the collecting system to ureters. Early ureteric bud division can lead to duplicate ureters. The mesenchyme forms the nephron proximal to the collection system of the Bowman's capsule through a mesenchymal-to-epithelial transition controlled mainly by the **PAX-2 gene**.

PAX-2 gene mutation and WT-1 can lead to an abnormal mesenchymal-to-epithelial transition, resulting in renal hypoplasia, agenesis, medullary cystic kidneys, nephroblastoma, etc. The kidney produces urine, which is the amniotic fluid in utero. This fluid pressure develops the fetal lungs. **Renal agenesis** is therefore associated with **Potter's Syndrome**, which is incompatible with life due to **oligohydraminos** and **lung hypoplasia**.

Telltale signs of renal developmental disease often include abnormal neonatal ears, colobomas (iris fissures), and **VACTERL**—vertebral anomalies, anal atresia, cardiac defects, trachea-esophageal fistulas, renal agenesis, and limb anomalies—*when at least three of these are present.*

If the *inferior poles of kidneys fuse*, they can form a **horseshoe kidney**. Horseshoe kidney ascent is often halted by the inferior mesenteric artery (IMA) and, although it may be of normal function, is often associated with **Turner's syndrome**.

Renal Physiology

Body Fluid Proportions:

Total body water (**TBW**) is *60%* of body weight. Antipyrine volume of distribution levels in the body can be used to estimate this.

One-third of TBW is intracellular fluid (**ICF**). (**TBW – ECF = ICF**)

Two-thirds of TBW is extracellular fluid (**ECF**). ECF volume can be determined by sulfate, inulin, or mannitol volumes of distribution as they are large and remain in the ECF compartment.

One-fourth of ECF is plasma. Determined using RISA (radioiodinated serum albumin).

Three-fourths is interstitial fluid (**IF**). (**ECF-Plasma=IF**)

Plasma osmolarity:

$$P_{osmo} = 2 \times Na^{+} (mEq/L) + (glucose\ mg/dL) / 18 + BUN\ (mg/dL) / 2.8)$$

When considering fluid shift, it is *important to consider the volume expansion or contractions in light of osmolarity changes*. (For example, iso-osmotic volume contraction (decrease in water volume with no change in osmolarity) is seen in diarrhea, hyperosmotic volume contraction (decrease in water volume and increase in osmolarity)is seen in sweating, hypoosmotic volume expansion is seen in SIADH, or hypoosmotic volume contraction is seen in adrenal insufficiency.)

The Nephron: Single functional unit with different parts

Corpuscle

Composed of **glomerulus capillaries** encased by the nephron tubular.

Bowman's capsule (site of filtration)

All but plasma proteins are filtered through **starling forces.**
Podocytes at the Bowman capsule have slits allowing filtration and **anionic glycoproteins**, which restrict the filtration of plasma proteins (*these are damaged in nephrotic syndrome*).
Sixty percent of calcium is filtered.

Proximal convoluted tubule (PCT)

Site of 100% glucose reabsorption through **Na+ / glucose transport** apically (tubule /lumen interface) and **GLUT transporters** basolaterally (tubule /peritubular capillary blood interface).

- $<$ **250 mg/dL** plasma glucose concentrations: complete reabsorption of glucose occurs
  - $>$ **250 mg/dL**: the carriers become saturated, and **glucosuria** will occur
  - $\geq$ **350 mg/dL**: complete saturation of the carriers, and **glucosuria** occurs

Amino acid: 100% reabsorbed
One hundred percent **carboxylate** reabsorbed via **transporters.**
Sixty-five percent of **Na+ / K+** and **HCO_3** reabsorption.
Urea: 50% reabsorbed *passively*
Phosphate: 85% reabsorbed via **Na+ / PO_4 cotransporter** (inhibited by parathyroid hormone). Fifteen percent of PO_4 is excreted in urine as no other segment reabsorbs PO_4.
Na+ is also absorbed by **Na+/H+ exchange**, which is directly linked to **HCO_3 reabsorption** (carbonic anhydrase inhibitors act on this).
Late PCT Na+ is reabsorbed with **Cl–**.
Ninety percent of calcium is reabsorbed at **PCT** and **thick ascending limb.**
Magnesium absorption is variable here.
Calcitriol is produced by **hydroxylation of $25(OH)_2D$ at 1 α position.**

Diuretic: **Acetazolamide** (a carbonic anhydrase inhibitor) acts on the early PCT. The major effect is **increased HCO_3 excretion**.

Loop of Henle

Urea secretion in thin descending limb by diffusion from the high concentration of urea in the **medullary interstitial fluid.**

Na+ / K+ / 2Cl- symporter, in the **thick ascending limb**, is impermeable to water (diluting segment).

Some **K+** diffuse back into the **tubule lumen**, leading to lumen **positive potential difference.**

Twenty-five percent of **Na+** reabsorbed.

Calcium/magnesium, especially in **thick ascending limb**. They *compete for reabsorption*; therefore, the higher concentration of one of them will lead to more excretion of the other.

HCO_3 reabsorbed in the **thick ascending limb.**

Diuretic: Loop diuretics (**furosemide, ethacrynic acid, and bumetanide**) inhibit the **Na+/K+/2CL- cotransport pump** on the thick ascending Loop of Henle. This leads to **NaCl / K+ / Ca2+ excretion**. Decreases the corticopapillary gradient. Bumetanide / ethacrynic acid can be used in sulfa allergy, unlike furosemide. **Furosemide IV** is half that of **the PO dose** in terms of **bioavailability**. **Torsemide** has a better **PO bioavailability** and could be used in **severe edema nonresponsive patients** as **an alternative to IV furosemide** dosing; however, it is hepatically eliminated and therefore should not be used in patients with **hepatic dysfunction**. **Continuous infusions** are associated with better **diuretic effect versus repeated boluses** and less **S/E** like **ototoxicity**; they can cause hypo- or hypernatremia, depending on volume status.

Distal tubule

Na+ / Cl– symporter, inhibited by thiazide diuretics.

Ten percent of **Na+** reabsorbed.
Impermeable to water—called the cortical diluting segment.
Calcium reabsorption in response to **PTH** by activating adenylate cyclase.
Magnesium reabsorption.
Impermeable to **urea.**

Diuretic: Thiazides (**chlorothiazide, hydrochlorothiazide**) inhibit the **Na+/Cl– cotransport** in **early distal tubule.** Leads to increased **NaCl / K+ excretion.** Decreases **calcium excretion.** No effect on the ability to concentrate urine. They are the most common cause of **drug induced hyponatremia.**

Diuretic: K+ sparing diuretics (**spironolactone, triamterene, amiloride**), act on **late distal tubule**, and collecting duct inhibition of **Na+ reabsorption, inhibition of K+ / H+ secretion** leads to weak **natriuresis** (mainly used for K+ sparing effect with loop or thiazides) and decreases **H+ excretion.**

Collecting tubule

Urea reabsorption at the medullary collecting tubule region. Impermeable to urea except at the inner medullary collecting ducts, where reabsorption of **urea** occurs due to **ADH stimulation** of the **UT1 diffusion transporter.**

Two cell types:

Principal: reabsorb Na+ and water and secrete K+.
Na+ reabsorption and **K+ secretion** via **aldosterone action** on amiloride sensitive Na+ channel aka **epithelial sodium channel (ENaC).**
(**ENaC** is upregulated in **cystic fibrosis** due to **defective CFTR gene**).
Only 2% of **Na reabsorption** is affected by **aldosterone.**

ADH causes water reabsorption via **V2 receptors and aquaporin regulation**. In the absence of ADH, it becomes essentially impermeable.
Alpha-Intercalated cells: reabsorb HCO_3 and secrete H+. H+ secretion and K + reabsorption by **H+ K+ ATpase** in **low K+ diet**.

Concentration of Urine

Mainly due to the corticopapillary osmotic gradient osmolarity of cortex 300 mOsmol/L to 1200 mOsmol/L at papilla. This is maintained by the countercurrent multiplication in the Loop of Henle (impervious ascending limb with 2Na / K / CL transportation) and urea recycling in the inner medullary collecting ducts (urea reabsorption in the inner medullary collecting system in response to ADH) and is maintained by countercurrent exchange in the vasa recta.

Acid Base Control

HCO_3 reabsorption

Mainly in early PCT.
Intracellular carbonic anhydrase catalyzes $\mathbf{CO_2 + H_2O \Leftrightarrow H_2CO_3 \Leftrightarrow HCO_3^- + H^+}$.
HCO_3^- then gets reabsorbed in blood, while **H+** is secreted back into **lumen** part of the Na+ / H+ exchange pump.
The **luminal H+** is involved in the same reaction as above, this time yielding **CO_2+ H_2O**, which diffuses back intracellularly.
This is affected by:

Filtered load: the more HCO_3, the more it will be excreted in urine.
PCO_2 levels: shifts the equilibrium in response to respiratory alkalosis or acidosis in an attempt to compensate.
ECF Volume: Volume expansion leads to less HCO_3 reabsorption. Volume contraction leads to higher HCO_3 reabsorption (**contraction alkalosis**).

Angiotensin II: stimulates the Na+ / H+ exchange pump and HCO_3 reabsorption.

Excretion of H^+

Luminal H^+ can either:

Combine with **HPO_4^{-2}** to form **titratable acid $H_2PO_4^-$**.
Combine with **NH_3 to form NH_4^+**. (NH_3 is formed from glutamine by renal cells and diffuses into lumen.)
Hyperkalemia inhibits **NH_3 synthesis**, which leads to decreased **H+ excretion** (renal tubular acidosis type 4, hyperaldosteronism).

Acid Base Disorders

Serum anion gap = (Na+) – (Cl–) + (HCO_3), normal is 12 mEq/L (range 8–16 mEq/L).

Normal anion gap—metabolic acidosis (Na/HCO_3—losses compensated by Cl–) (BAD FRCSI): , B-blocker, acid ingestion, diarrhea, GI fistulas, pancreatic disease, renal tubular acidosis, carbonic anhydrase inhibitors, , spironolactone, ileostomy.

Increased anion gap metabolic acidosis: (MUD PILES) unaccounted for serum anions increased to replace HCO_3 (methanol, uremia, diabetic ketoacidosis, paracetamol toxicity, infection, lactic acidosis, ethanol, salicylates).

Cl– responsive metabolic alkalosis: Urine Cl is less than fifteen, vomiting, diuretics, pyloric stenosis, laxatives.

Cl– resistant metabolic alkalosis: Urine Cl is greater than fifteen, severe Mg/K deficiency **(diuretic abuse)**, Conns syndrome, Bartter syndrome, tobacco chewing, licorice consumption.

Other Functions of the Kidney

Gluconeogenesis

Renal cortex can account for up to 50% of **gluconeogenesis** during fasting.

Primary organ is the **liver**.

Mainly substrates for glucose production are from:

lactate → pyruvate → glucose (Cori cycle)

glycerol (fatty acid breakdown) →pyruvate → glucose

glutamate →TCA cycle → pyruvate →glucose

The renal medulla is not involved in gluconeogenesis.

Erythropoiesis

Erythropoietin production by **interstitial fibroblasts** close to peritubular capillaries and PCT in response to **hypoxemia**, stimulating **bone marrow erythropoiesis**.

Prostaglandins Secretions

Homeostatic Mechanisms

Renin-Angiotensin System

Renin released in response to:

Decreased perfusion pressure sensed by the juxtaglomerular apparatus (**JGA**).

Increased sodium sensed by the **macula densa**.

Increased sympathetic stimulation (β-1 adrenergic receptor stimulation), mainly found in proximal tubular epithelium and renal artery smooth muscles.

β-1—**adrenaline** coupled to **Gs surface protein**, which activates **adenylyl cyclase** →increases **cAMP** production, which activates **Protein Kinase A**, which **phosphorylates myosin light chain kinase** leading to **smooth muscle relaxation**. Also causes cardiac muscle contraction and glycogenolysis.

Hyperkalemia.

Renin release inhibited by:

Hypokalemia.

Renin circulating in blood converts **angiotensinogen** (produced the liver) to **angiotensin I.**

Angiotensin converting enzyme (**ACE**) in the lung cleaves angiotensin I to **form angiotensin II.**

Angiotensin II:

Net change is increased in **BP** with eventual restoration of renal perfusion via:

Aldosterone adrenal cortex release, which causes:

Distal convoluted tubule Na+/K+-ATPase transporter activation → water and sodium reabsorption and K+ excretion.

Na+/H+ exchanger activation ↑H+ excretion and **metabolic alkalosis.**

Antidiuretic hormone release from the **posterior pituitary,** which:

Also released in **high blood osmolality.**

Causes **water reabsorption** in **collecting ducts.**

Acts on **V2 receptors** → increased **cAMP** and **intracellular calcium** → increases **collecting tubules aquaporins channels transcription.**

Acts as a **vasoconstrictor.**

Increases cardiac afterload and therefore work.

Decreases renal perfusion and therefore urinary loss.

Sympathetic activation, causing increased heart rate and cardiac output.

Hypothalamus reflex activation of thirst.

Atrial Natriuretic Peptide

Release by atrial wall distension from volume overload:

Inhibits **Na+** and **water reabsorption** by inhibiting ADH effects.

Vasodilation of **afferent arterioles** (lesser extent vasoconstriction of efferent arterioles).
Inhibits **renin** and **aldosterone** production.

Ethanol

Inhibits **vasopressin release** by blocking **calcium dependent channels**, net effect is diuresis.

Cortisol

Inhibits **ADH secretion.**

Prostaglandin E2 and I2, bradykinin, nitric oxide, and dopamine cause **renal arteriolar vasodilation** and increased renal blood flow.

Glomerular Filtration Rate (GFR)

GFR most accurately and reliably measured by **isotope clearance (Iothalamate clearance)**, accepted 80 ml/min/m^2 (adjusted by age and not widely available).
CrCl: Twenty-four hours urine collection (tends to **overestimate**).
eGFR: using modified in diet and renal Disease (**MDRD**) or **Cockcroft-Gault** (tends to underestimate but better than CrCl).
Average of the **MDRD + CrCl** is better than any of the individual tests (CG / MDRD / CrCl).
Controlled by the efferent limb.
Stages of **chronic kidney disease** (**CKD**) as measured by **GFR:**

- **Stage 1: Normal, GFR > 90 ml/min.**
- **Stage 2: Mild CKD, GFR 60–89 ml/min.**
- **Stage 3: Moderate CKD, GFR 30–59 ml/min.**
- **Stage 4: Severe CKD, GFR 15–29 ml/min.**
- **Stage 5: End stage CKD, GFR < 15 ml/min.**

Energy and Fuel Metabolism in the Kidney

Renal Oxygen Consumption

The **kidney** receives 25% of **cardiac output**—greatest percentage.

It has the second highest per weight oxygen delivery to an organ (3,500 μmol/ min / 100 g), the first being the heart.

The **renal vein** has **high oxygen tension**, due to the overall low oxygen extraction; despite this, the kidney also has the second highest oxygen consumed per weight of any organ, second to the heart.

Oxygen consumption increases as a function of **renal blood flow**. As GFR increases, tubules are at increased work with solute shifts—requiring **Na+/K+-ATPase**.

Sodium Reabsorption

Is the major **energy expenditure source** of the kidney.

Sodium absorption is **extremely energy efficient** in the kidney.

Clinically, 28–33 moles of sodium are reabsorbed per one mole of oxygen consumed.

However, using accepted stoichiometry, one mole of oxygen results in six moles of ATP. Three moles of sodium are reabsorbed per one mole of ATP, which results mathematically in eighteen moles of sodium per one mole of oxygen consumed. This suggested that there are more efficient processes that may not be directly related to ATP consumption or multiply the efficiency of the ATP effect that allows for efficient sodium consumption.

Complete sodium pump inhibition only decreases sodium reabsorption by 50%.

Basal Oxygen Consumption

Oxygen consumption by processes that are independent of sodium reabsorption—hard to calculate.

Up to 25% of this can be stimulated by **gluconeogenesis**.

Oxygen distribution in the kidney is **nonhomogeneous**.

Cytochrome a/a3 (electron transport chain) is oxidized at 98% in well oxygenated organs, but it's only 60% in the kidney, which suggests it works almost at the brink of hypoxia.

Bumetanide inhibition in the ascending limb of the Loop of Henle increases the **cytochrome a/a3 oxidization** in the outer medulla.

There is a significant drop in oxygen gradient like a countercurrent of oxygen, the further out from the cortex closer to the papilla. The greatest drop occurs at the level of the outer medulla into the inner medulla. There is little to no aerobic metabolism in the inner medulla, which is mirrored by the decrease in mitochondrial distribution.

Metabolic Substrate in the Kidney

Cortex: **Short and long fatty acids, ketone bodies, lactate,** and some **amino acids**

Outer medulla**: Succinate / lactate**

Inner medulla: **Glucose** preferred due to hypoxia

The preferred rank of energy source is: lactate, free fatty acids, citrate, and pyruvate. (This is hard to account for, in in-vitro tissue—there is no to minimal pump activity, while in in-vivo tissue it is hard to differentiate substrate concentration related to consumption vs those produced).

Glycolysis

Mainly from **glucose** when there are very low glycogen stores. Rate cannot be accurately depicted but based on glycolysis enzymes distribution in the nephron. They are predominant in the **distal nephron**.

Key enzymes being **hexokinase, phosphofructokinase (PFK),** and **pyruvate kinase.**

Papilla are thought to work mainly through **anaerobic glycolysis** condition, especially if work is increased (e.g., during osmotic diuresis).

Papilla preferably use **glucose** even with an abundance of pyruvate lactate.

Hexose Monophosphate Shunt

About 10% of **glucose metabolism.**

Pathway providing a rich source of **NADPH.**

Thought to have a role in renal synthetic processes (renin production and in compensatory renal hypertrophy after a unilateral nephrectomy).

Its actions are stimulated by **diabetes** and inhibited by **hypertrophy.**

Sorbitol Pathway

Glucose is converted to **sorbitol** via **aldose reductase.**

Abundant throughout the kidney.

Activity is increased by **hyperosmotic stress, ADH hormone, dehydration,** and **hypernatremia,** thereby accumulating in the inner medulla and allowing water retention.

Sorbitol conversion to **fructose** via sorbitol dehydrogenase is needed in **hypo-osmotic states.**

Renal Gluconeogenesis

Mainly in the **proximal tubule.**

Rich in key enzymes: **glucose-6-phosphatase, fructose 1,6-diphosphatase (F1,6DP), phosphoenolpyruvate carboxykinase (PEPCK).**

The kidney contributes up to 25% of **gluconeogenesis** in normal conditions and **50%** during starvation or diabetes.

Stimulated by **metabolic acidosis** (DKA, exercise, fasting) and inhibited by **metabolic alkalosis** (bicarbonate administration).

F1, DP, and PEPCK activities are also stimulated by glucocorticoids, Norepinephrine, PTH, and Vitamin D; it is inhibited by calcitonin.

It has a reciprocal relation to sodium reabsorption.

Na+/K+-ATPase inhibition, and therefore sodium inhibition, stimulates gluconeogenesis.

Lactate Metabolism

Lactate dehydrogenase is abundant along the **nephron**. It is used to convert **lactate** to **pyruvate**.

Lactate is the mainly consumed part of the gluconeogenesis pathway.

Lactate supports sodium reabsorption.

Lipid metabolism

Long and short fatty acids are believed to support sodium reabsorption.

Immunology

Primary Lymphoid Organs

Bone, liver, and thymus

Secondary Lymphoid Organs

Spleen and lymph nodes

Innate Immune System

Nonspecific, nonmemory-based immunity, mainly based on inflammation and complement system activations

Cells: Phagocytes—**PMNs, macrophages, natural killer** (NK) **cells, mast cells, basophils,** and **eosinophils**

Adaptive Immune System

T cells: specific action through interactions with nonself on antigen processing cells (APC) →**cell-mediated immunity**

B cells: antibody-based interactions to nonself → **humoral immunity**

Both processes (cellular and humoral):

- Use **innate cells** to execute the complete response.
- Memory response to specific antigens.
- Primary response is slower than innate immunity, and secondary response is usually much faster and aggressive.

Humoral Immunity

Matures in bone and develops **B-cell receptors (BCR).**

BCR is a **membrane-bound antibody** that is specific to an antigen.

Mature B cells migrate to **lymph nodes** and **lymphatic organs.**

They act as Antigen Presenting Cells (**APC**) to **T cells**; they produce inflammatory cytokines, and some subpopulations (**B$_{reg}$**) **secrete IL-10,** which modulates the immune response. Upon encountering a matching antigen in its native form (not processed), and **T$_H$2 cells** have activated it **(IL-4)** → **B cells** will divide:

Clonal expansion into **active plasma cells** (produce antigen-specific antibodies), which live for two to three days.

Memory cells (10%)—responsible for **IgG secondary future responses** to the same antigen if encountered.

Antibodies

IgM

Most common (MC) Ab (antibody) in the spleen. Lacking after a splenectomy and as result patients at risk of overwhelming postsplenectomy infection (OPSI).

Responsible for the primary antibody response—indicates **acute infection / rejection**, etc.

The largest antibody—does not cross the placenta.

Pentamer (ten binding sites).

Activates complement.

Opsonization for phagocytosis.

IgG

MC antibody overall (75%).

Activates complement (takes two **IgGs**).

Opsonization for phagocytosis.

Can cross the placenta.

Secondary response to antigen.

This leads to antibody-mediated cellular toxicity via innate cells stimulation through an Fc receptor on them.

Associated with **Type 2 (hyperacute rejection)** and **Type 3 hypersensitivity**.

IgA

Mucosal immunity.

Secreted by **plasma cells** and then gets taken up by epithelial cells and secreted in mucosal luminal surfaces.
Prevents pathogen adherence to the epithelium by coating them.

IgD

Membrane-bound receptor on **B cells**.
Expressed only when B cells are mature.

IgE

Type 1 hypersensitivity and parasite infections.
Binds to **mast cells** and **basophils** via **Fc portion**.

Cell-mediated immunity

T cells mature in the thymus through negative and positive selection.

T cells (**CD4**) differentiate into four main helper subpopulations and one regulatory subpopulation.

Effector T_H cells:

T_H1 cells: target macrophages (bactericidal) via IFNγ. **Responsible for rejection**. Differentiates mainly due to IL-12.

Secretes **IFNγ, TNFα** and **lymphotoxin** → activate **macrophages,** damages **graft endothelium,** induces **IgG production** by **B cells** and **CD8+ T cell** to **cytotoxic cells. Target drug anti-IL-12p20. Ustekinumab used in psoriasis treatment**

T_H2 cells: Responsible for **allergic reactions** and **rejection**. Differentiates due to IL-4.

It produces mainly IL-4 in addition to many other IL that enhance particular isotype Ab production by B cells. It activates **eosinophils, mast cells,** and **basophils**. Less potent than TH1 but has some dampening role to TH1 through IL-10.

T_H17 cell: subpopulation particular at responding to **fungal infections**. Induced by **IL-6** and **IL-23**.

It produces **IL-17**, a neutrophil chemoattractant, and other stromal cells in the graft. Leads to the development of tertiary lymphoid tissue. **Anti-IL-17 Ab, called secukinumab, for treatment of psoriasis and rheumatoid arthritis**

T_{FH} cell: Follicular helper cells play an important role in **B cell Ab production.** They differentiate in response to IL-21. They migrate to B-cell follicles in secondary tissue and induce activated B-cell differentiation to plasma cells via CD40L-CD40 interaction and through the production of IL-4 + IL-21.

T_{reg} cell: differentiates due to IL-2 and TGFβ. It produces **IL-10,** which aids at dampening rejection.

Memory T cells:

Involved in **secondary immune response**. Most effector cells undergo activation-induced cell death. However, some cells in response to IL-7 and IL-15 will differentiate into memory cells. Their response is more potent and specific to alloantigens. Often not requiring costimulatory (signal 2) pathway (B7-CD28 inhibition is not effective) There is also a resurgence of their level when recovering from lymphopenia, which explains why thymoglobulin and Campath have on average high memory cells versus nondepleted regimens

Two types of memory cells:

T_{CM} cells (central memory): have **CCR7 receptor** and have **secondary lymphoid** and **nonlymphoid** presence.

T_{EM} cells (effector memory): have **CXCR3 receptor**, have predominant **nonlymphoid presence**, and have a more potent response.

Cytotoxic T cells (CD8+):

Directly attack MHC-1 nonself cells via perforins and granzymes.

Enhanced via IL-2 and TNFγ production of T helper cells—inhibited via calcineurin inhibitors.

Natural Killer Cells:

Activated by IL-2, but their response is independent of the TCR-MHC recognition.

Attack cells lacking **MHC** or have **low expression** of MHC.

Attack **Ab-antigen complexes** (Fc receptor).

Hypersensitivity Reaction:

Type 1: Immediate hypersensitivity—**anaphylaxis / allergy** provoked by re-exposure to **antigen.**

IgE-mediated response of **mast cells** (in tissues) / **basophils** (in blood).

Type 2: Antibody-dependent cytotoxicity—**ITP, HUS, hyperacute rejection**.

IgG or **IgM**.

Antigen-antibody complex bound to innate immunity cells via Fc portion.

Complement activation.

Type 3: Immune complex deposit—**serum sickness** (*thymoglobulin / ATGAM*).

Antigen-antibody (**IgG**) complex deposits on **vessel walls** and induces **inflammation**.

Type 4: Chronic rejection—delayed hypersensitivity.

Antibody independent.

T cells detect tissues as foreign and are activated to **T_H1 cells—tissue destruction**.

Complement Activation:

Classic pathway:

Activated:

Antigen-Ab complex (**IgG / IgM**).

Direct pathogen binding to **C1**.

First step is C1 formation.

C1, C2, and **C4** are specific to classic pathway.

Alternate Pathway:

Activation:

First step is **C3** activation by **bacteria, endotoxins,** etc.

Factors B, D, and properdin are specific to alternate pathways.

Convergence of both pathways at **C3**. Both pathways need **Mg^{2+}**.

Results in:

membrane attack complex C5b-C9b—cell lysis

C3b-C4b—opsonization

C3a-C5a—chemotaxis

HLA and MHC

Human Leukocyte Antigen (HLA) is a gene complex coded on the short arm of **Chromosome 6.**
It codes for the **major histocompatibility (MHC)** protein, which is crucial in discriminating self from non-self.

HLA Class 1 Codes:

Classical: HLA A, B, and C code for the heavy chains (α). Expressed under physiologic stress.

Nonclassical: minor genes HLA E, F, and G. The expression of these is restricted to specific tissue.

HLA-like genes: MICA and MIC.
Expresses MHC 1 molecules, which can present peptides processed from within the cells (e.g., viruses' peptides).

MHC class 1—is expressed on all nucleated cells. Interacts directly and activates and controls the function of **CD8 cytotoxic T cells.**

Nonclassical and **HLA**-like genes code for **ligands** to receptors that control the natural killer activation.
HLA class 1 is single chain with five domains.

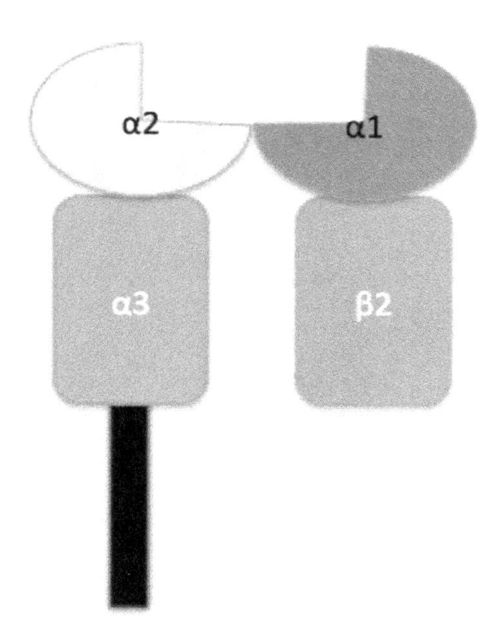

HLA Class 2:

Classical: code heavy (α) and light (β) chains for **HLA DP / DQ / DR** (α chain of DR is the only one that is not polymorphic).

Nonclassical: class 2 HLA are DM and DO. Code for **heterotetrameric complexes** that are involved in **peptide exchanges** onto the classical Class II molecules.

MHC class 2: expressed on **APC** (dendritic / B cells / macrophages), endothelial activated cells in inflammation—expresses antigens from outside the cell (e.g., phagocytosis of bacterial proteins).

Interact with **CD4 T_H cells**, which:

Stimulates the **B cell antibody response** via **T_H 2 cells (IL-4)**.

Stimulates the **macrophages response (IFNγ)**.

HLA Class 2 are two chains with four domains each.

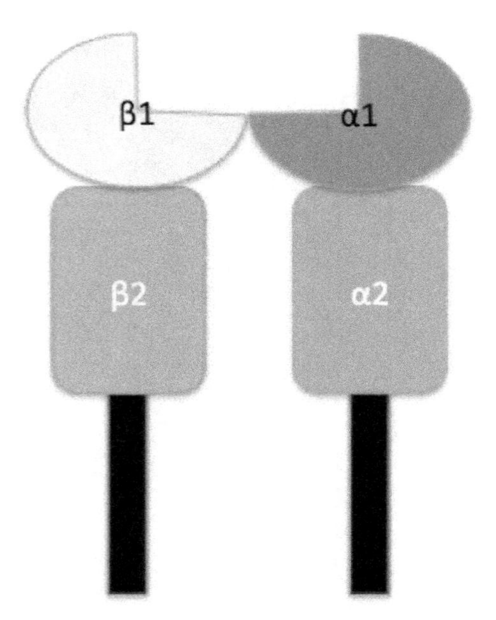

HLA Class 3:

Codes the complement pathway, **tumor necrosis factors,** and **heat shock proteins.**

- **HLA A, B,** and **DR** are used in **kidney allocation**. There is tremendous **allele variation** and combination but also some that is racially or geographically more common.
- **HLA matching** is more crucial for success than increased cold time.
- The most common **HLA antigen** is **A2** (50% of populations around the world), expressed as **HLA-A*02:01** in 96% of Caucasian ancestry but mainly as **HLA-A*02:06** in Hispanic and Chinese ancestry.

- **HLA** matching not done for liver transplant—only **ABO matching**.

MHC genes are inherited in Mendelian fashion, but recombination can occur on a locus, and unaccounted minor genes can also initiate rejections if not considered.

Patient X: HLA A / B / DR
Paternal copy: A2, B8, DR4
Maternal copy: A1, B44, DR15

- The offspring would inherit one haplotype, either his paternal or maternal original copy. So they (parent and son) would be one haplotype match, and genetically those alleles of the haplotypes would theoretically be identical. This would be impossible to determine if the patients were unrelated, as we would not know how the haplotypes are connected, and so we only know the phenotype of the individual (i.e., referring to patient X: HLA A2, A1, B8, B44, DR4 and DR15). The degree off commonness between donor and recipient is then described as the three-antigen match or mismatch.
- Certain HLA phenotype occur more frequently in populations, which suggests the existence on a common locus due to some positive selection bias (e.g., the HLA A1-B8 haplotype exits above predicted incidence [8%]).
- Alloantibodies are divided into:
  - Private group (i.e., they share an epitope that is specific to HLA molecule).
  - Public group: they are an epitope that is shared by more than one allele. Most common example in BW6 / BW4 (aka cross reactive groups CREGs).
    - Identifying short tandem repeats can differentiate between fraternal (need

immunosuppression) versus identical twins (no need for immunosuppression).

ABO Blood Compatibility:

Blood group AB—(has no Ab to A or B)—universal recipient
Blood group O—(has Ab to A and B)—universal donor

ABO incompatible transplants have been performed (*see desensitization chapter page 95*) but at increased cost and risk. They are often done for living donors or kidney paired exchange programs, allowing for desensitization protocols to be performed electively before the transplants.
A_2 (20% of the white population has reduced A antigen expression on graft endothelium, allowing for their transplantation into O and B recipients).

HLA Matching

Identifying HLA Antibodies in Donors

Complement Dependent Cytotoxic (CDC)

- Lymphocytes and antigen mixed from recipient serum with a rabbit serum (source of complement) versus donor T cell / B cell.
- Activation and lysis are seen on staining.
- IgM antibodies can interfere with testing, especially if patients have autoimmune disease, so to enhance the specificity to the IgG, either prolong the complement incubation or add antihuman globulin (AHG).
- Positive crossmatch is a contraindication for transplant.

Flow Cytometry (FCXM)

- Tests patient sera for an anti-CD3 (pan T-cell marker) and anti-CD19 / anti-CD20 (B cell markers) conjugate with fluorescent dyes (PE phycoerythrin or PerCP peridinin chlorophyll protein)
- The degree of yellow-green fluorescence represents the degree of T cell / B cell antibody titer. It can detect very low levels of circulating antibodies.
- Positive FCXM does not mean a transplant is contraindicated. It is associated with higher risk of early acute rejection and lower one-year graft survival, especially if associated with sensitization history and older and uncertain kidney quality grafts.
- There are cases where CDC was negative and FCXM was positive that had an uneventful transplant, but it is crucial to look at sensitization history and HLA solid

phase assay antibodies before considering a false positive test.
- Pronase treatment of donor cells can help differentiate false positive tests related to the binding of nonspecific antibodies without affecting HLA molecules.

Virtual Crossmatch

- Uses previously inputted HLA data of patient from solid phase assay and complete HLA donor information to identify compatibility using a computer algorithm.
- Dependent on accuracy of inputted information and up-to-date patient HLA.
- Can significantly decrease cold time.
- Recommend waiting on crossmatches for highly sensitized patients as missed input, unacceptable antigens, or incomplete donor information can ultimately result in a positive crossmatch.
- In some cases adding every HLA antigen a patient has as unacceptable can in some practices adjust the chances of the patient's likelihood of transplants, especially if there is no uniform MFI level that can be used as a cutoff for a crossmatch, especially if the CDC was negative, thereby changing a patient's CPRA.
- Good practice is to test a patient's HLA every three months. Patients without an updated HLA, especially if sensitized or at high risk of routine transfusions, can acquire antibodies that may be missed.

Solid-Phase Assay

Purified or engineered HLA antigens to identify HLA antibodies.

Three types:

- **Mixed bead:** has a mix of donor HLA class 1 and 2 antigens, least sensitive, used to screen blood donors for TRALI.

- **Phenotype bead:** mixture of HLA antigens and is similar to testing an individual's lymphocytes. However, antigens may be masked by overactive sera, blocking it, leading to poor specificity.
- **Single antigen bead:** detects reactivity to single antigens and some common alleles used to characterize HLA in highly sensitized patients.
- There is no established mean fluorescence intensity (MFI) level that correlates with a positive CDC crossmatch. There is a probability of a positive flow cytometry with an MFI greater than five thousand but may be set differently for different antigens—CREGs or highly sensitized patients.
- Some antigens like DP or DQ have a large number of epitopes, which are hard to be tested on a single bead test, such that in some instances even when DP / DQ is coded as an antibody, their significance may or may not be as true for e.g. *DPB1*40:01 is very different to the DPB1*105:01.*

Molecular Typing and Identifying Recipient HLA Genes and Antigens

Used to identify **specific alleles through PCR.**

Three types:

Sequence-specific oligonucleotide probe (SSOP) a form of enzyme-linked or fluorescent markers read on a flow cytometer or Luminex machine of group alleles or HLA antigen (i.e., only identifies the antigen or allele group, not the genetic code of it).

Sequence Specific Primers (SSP): use agarose gel to separate the allele specific primers PCR by size. Also does not identify the exact allele (low to moderate resolution).

Sequence Based Typing (SBT): can identify the exact allele of an antigen by detecting variance in nucleotide. Considered high resolution testing.

- Low and intermediate resolution are used in solid organ transplants.
- High resolution is more specific and is used in bone marrow transplant.

Antibody Detection and Quantification:
- Cell based—CDC / flow cytometry.
- Solid phase (identify the peripheral molecule)—ELISA / Luminex/ Flow cytometry.
- PRA: Panel Reactive Antibody, is the percentage of a population an individual will react to for e.g. PRA of 16% means an individual has antibody against 16% of the population. Currently 20% receive special ranking. Ninety-seven percent priority, 98% local power pull, 99% regional power pull, 100% national power pull.

Role is to identify "acceptable" mismatches.
- Prevent hyperacute rejection.
- AMR risk assessment:
  - Some antibodies are amnestic and then erupt if transplant occurs, even though it was not detected in a CDC test.
    - Risk factors include:
      - Pregnancy (40% sensitized, higher for multiparous)
      - Transfusions
      - Previous transplants (75% sensitized)
    - Chronic rejection due to continuous exposure to DSA, which may appear posttransplant.

Transplant Immunology

T cell receptors (TCR) bind to MHC I (all nucleated cells).
MHC 1 cells with allopeptides will cause T cells to react.
Therefore, T cell should be able to bind to self without activating self.

Thymic Selection (aka Central Tolerance):

- **Negative selection:** Cells that bind to APC with high affinity will die, but those with low affinity will survive. This is imperfect and hence autoimmunity.
- **Positive selection:** TCR bind to thymic epithelial cells—the affinity of which will determine if the cell survives. The ability to detect antigen in the context of self MHC is positively selected.

Peripheral tolerance:

- Maintained by T_{reg} and B_{reg} cells that suppress T cells and B cells or cause states of anergy or exhaustion. Key cytokines produced by them are IL-10 and TGFβ. **Anergy** is a state of unresponsiveness due to a lack of costimulatory response (signal 2 pathway). **Exhaustion** is a state when repeated stimulation leads to the expression of inhibitory molecules like PD-1, which keeps T cells hypo- or under responsive.

Tolerance: Host with intact immunity that does not destroy his allograft. Not guaranteed by current immunosuppression regimens, but the most promising is when the central tolerance is achieved by ablation of recipient immune system and then reconstituting it at the central level to incorporate graft alloantigen recognizing cells (often will require also donor bone marrow transplantation), therefore creating a transient or permanent chimeric immune system that does not reject donor organs.

Accessory molecules like CD 4 bind to the TCR / protein and MHC II (APC) to stabilize the weak noncovalent bond.

CD 8 helps stabilize MHC I molecules bond.

But foreignness does not always lead to interaction. Pregnant women don't attack their fetus—but would if they had a fetus organ transplanted into them after delivery. This is due to the fact that T-cell activation is a bell-curve shape with optimal interaction at the center of the curve leading to activation. This center is when optimization occurs due to optimal cytokines / inflammation, etc. Therefore from a surgical point, the greater the reperfusion injury, the higher the T-cell risk of activation; also that's how autoimmunity could develop even if the T cells have been engineered for self-recognition.

Costimulatory Proteins—Regulating T-Cell Response:

- **CD 28 Binding to B7:**
  - Leads to activation of T cells.
  - Upregulation of CD 152 (aka CTLA4)—binds B7 with higher affinity and competes with CD 28 and leads to a downregulatory response to T cells.
- **CD 40 Ligand / CD 154:**
  - Binds CD 40 on APC.
  - Increases MHC expression and B7.

Therefore, when discussing immunity in transplant and rejection:

- We naturally have a higher percentage of precursor cells that are not adapted to the new organ antigens.
- The reperfusion of that organ allows for APC interaction and specific chemotaxis to the offending organ or tissue.

- The organ susceptibility will determine the response too, as a liver will be able to tolerate higher number of T cells attacks versus sinoatrial node of the heart.

Alloantigens:

- Foreign molecules between genetically different individuals of the same species.
- Most important in transplant HLA are HLA-A, B, and DR with great variance, but other HLA are still important.

Donor derived APC and cellular debris migrate to the spleen and secondary lymphoid tissue and are processed to T cells, resulting in them being primed for activation or activation.

- **Allorecognition by T Cells:**
  - **Direct Pathway:** Donor APC directly interacts with T cells.
    - The precursor frequency (number of naive T cells that will recognize it as foreign) is higher (1–10% of the recipient T cell population).
      - CD4 recognizes MHC II of donor cells.
      - CD8 recognizes MHC I of donor cells.
  - **Indirect Pathway:** debris processed by recipient APC presented to T cells.
    - Precursor frequency is one hundred times weaker than the direct.
      - CD4 cell recognize the allopeptides part of MHC-II of the recipient.
      - CD 8 cells recognize allopeptides on MHC-I.
  - Both CD4 and CD8 cells are able to independently cause rejection.
    - CD4 cells:
      - Help full activation of CD8.
      - It can cause direct cytotoxicity by cytokine release or Fas ligand expression.
      - More susceptible to co-stimulation blockade than CD8 cells.

- CD8 cells—conventionally are thought of as more cytotoxic via perforins and granzyme expression, which are also expressed by NK cells.
  - Perforin allows granzymes entry into target cells.
  - Granzymes activate the→ caspase pathway, which leads to apoptosis.
- Antibody mediated cytotoxicity.
  - Alloantibody binds the alloantigen.
    - Leads to complement activation.
    - Binds the Fc portion of the effector cell that ends up causing phagocytosis or cell lysis.

Transplant Pharmacology

Immunosuppression:

Individuals respond differently to immunosuppression. Immunosuppression is an ambiguous term as some immunosuppression may actually promote immunity through costimulatory receptors and responses and vice versa.

Target Signals:

- **Signal 1:** TCR—response to HLA-peptide complex→ CD3 complex activation. Results in activation of phospholipase C-γ (PLC-γ).
  - PLC catalyzes (membrane lipid) PIP_2 → DAG + IP_3.
    - IP3 → (↑Intracellular calcium) triggers the calcineurin pathway.
    - DAG → activates protein kinase C (PKC) and mitogen-activated protein kinase (MAP).
    - PKC + MAP + calcineurin pathway → activate transcription factors (NFAT, NFkB, AP-1) → code activation of cytokine genes → T cell proliferation and differentiation.
  - Calcineurin inhibitors like tacrolimus and cyclosporine:
    - Inhibit the calcineurin pathway.
    - Potent T cell activation (naive and memory).
    - Is not dependent on antigenicity or specificity.
- **Signal 2:** Receptors or co-stimulator blockades that augment the TCR response (e.g., CD28, CTLA4, CD154 [CD40L]). They are only effective if signal one is activated. Failure to provide a second signal results in

aborted activation → T cell death or anergy (refractoriness to stimulation to antigen). Costimulatory molecules upregulated, allowing for amplification of T cells exposed to the antigen.

- **Integrins LFA-1** and **CD2** provide initial transient adhesion between the T cell and allopresenting cell. TCR changes the integrins conformation and increases its affinity. LFA-1 and CD2 deliver intracellular signaling.
    - Target drugs: anti-LFA-1 (Efalizumab), anti-CD2 (Alefacept).
- **B7-CD28:** CD28 on T cells binds to B7.1 (CD80) and B7.2 (CD86). TCR must be engaged too. Augments the above PLC-γ pathway.
    - Target drug: Belatacept (CTLA4-Ig) inhibits B7 engagement of CD28. Used as an alternative to CIN.
- **CD40-CD154:** CD154 AKA (CD40L) expressed on activated CD4+ T cells. CD 40 is expressed on B cells. The interaction between them → B cell isotype switching (the more effective IgG is produced instead of IgM) + B7 molecule upregulation (see above).
    - Target drugs: anti-CD154 (not used due to thromboembolic events as it's expressed on PLTs). Anti-CD40L in works.
- Only useful for naive T cells: they are dependent on costimulatory pathways unlike memory cells that are not.
- Preserves specificity, as TCR is still available for APC.

- **Signal 3:** Cytokine pathways that augment immune responses (e.g., IL-2 pathways action) → anti-Tac molecules, anti-CD52, anti-JAK stat pathway, and mTOR pathways → affects T-cell proliferation and differentiation. Affects other immune cells.
    - IL-2: activated T cells, express a third α chain to the normal β, γ IL-2 receptors (IL-2R). This α (AKA CD25) chain enhances the IL-2R affinity by one thousand →

clonal T cell expansion. Γ chain receptor activation is through the Janus Kinase (JAK) pathway

- Target drug: Anti-CD25 AKA basiliximab (weak induction) may be because other cytokines have a role also in this pathway. Anti-γ chain receptor → causes severe lymphopenia, genetically absent in severe combined immunodeficiency (SCID).
- Late inhibitor after activation has occurred but prevents its amplification.

- **Signal 4:** Adhesion molecules like CD2 pathway.
  - Interferes with cell trafficking of activated cells.
  - More effective on memory / active cells as they express more adhesion molecules.

Use of Biological Agents

- **Monoclonal** (Single cell line, reactive to a single epitope) versus **polyclonal:** Combination of Ig directed to a specific antigen, each identifying a different epitope (thymoglobulin).
- **Depleting** (All polyclonal) versus **nondepleting** (most monoclonal).
- **Humanized** (*Zu* stem, i.e., Dacli*zu*mab, three limited murine complementary determining regions on the variable region; the rest are all human IgG) versus **chimeric** (recombinant combination—variable region is all murine but the rest is human IgG, *xi* stem, e.g., Basili*xi*mab) versus **murine** (severe inflammatory response and production of HAMA—human anti-mouse antibodies).

Historically, produced via fusion of myeloma cells and spleen cells of an immunized mouse with a specific antigen. Now it's recombinant engineering.

Monoclonals Used:

- Induction, acute rejection, desensitization treatment.
- Types:
  - **Muromonab-CD3:**
    - Also known as OKT3, no longer in market since 2010. Murine Ab, HAMA with first use. Strong Cytokine release syndrome. Used in steroid-resistant rejection, sometimes off-label induction. Also was used in some desensitization protocols.
  - **Basiliximab:**
    - Also known as Simulect, (nondepleting), chimeric, anti-CD25 abIL-2 receptor Ab, 20 mg infusions (first on day zero (preop), second on postop day four),

long half-life (seven days). Used for induction. **MC Monoclonal** used.

- **Daclizumab:**
  - Also known as Zenapax, Humanized, nondepleting, long half-life, IL-2 Ab. Induction agent, no longer used since 2009. Alternative use in treatment of multiple sclerosis is being studied.
- **Alemtuzumab:**
  - Also known as Campath 1H, (**depleting**) humanized, T / B / macrophages and natural killer cells bind CD-52 receptor. Single induction dose (30 mg) can be given peripherally "off-label," but is gaining popularity. Used also for **B cell CLL treatment**.
  - Not superior to Thymoglobulin. But lower rejection versus basiliximab.
  - Increased risk of rejection when used in protocols that also include early steroid withdrawal.
  - Profound and prolonged lymphopenia (can last up to a year) compared to thymo, and therefore lower maintenance immunosuppressive doses can be used; however, quoted infectious risks are equivalent.
- **Rituximab:**
  - Anti CD20, on B cells, chimeric, monoclonal. Used for recurrent FSGS, acute humoral rejection, desensitization, to treat lymphoproliferative disease (PTLD), Non-Hodgkin's and some autoimmune conditions (e.g., ITP). Does not affect plasma cells. B cell recovery takes six months after administration.
  - Needs adequate premedication and slow initiation with dose incrementation.
  - Standard dose 375 mg/m^2.
  - Rare PML association and deaths with active Hep B.
- **Eculizumab:**
  - Also known as Soliris, humanized, monoclonal ab, inhibits C5a/b cleavage and MAC formation. FDA

approved for atypical HUS and PNH. Has been used to treat complement-mediated microvascular damage associated with AMR. Most expensive agent. Given at day zero (1200 mg), day one (900 mg) and weekly (900 mg) for the first month / biweekly (1200 mg) for the first month and then monthly. Is associated with meningococcal infection, and patients need vaccination two weeks prior to its elective use. Prophylactic use of ciprofloxacin.

- **Bortezomib:**
    - Also known as Velcade, proteasomal inhibitor (20S subunit) used for multiple myeloma. It has a proapoptopic effect on plasma cells (G2-M cell cycle).
    - Suppresses T cell function. Therefore potential to treat ACR and ABMR.
    - Adverse effects include peripheral neuropathy and thrombocytopenia.
- **Belatacept:**
    - Also known as Nulojix, monoclonal fusion protein containing transmembrane protein (CTLA-4) attached to an IG1 FC portion.
    - CTLA 4 linked to FC IgG → inhibits the costimulation of CD-28 and B7 involved on T cell activation.
    - FDA approved as maintenance + MMF and prednisone. (alternative to tacrolimus).
        - IV (10 mg/kg) POD 1, 5, week 2, week 4, monthly thereafter.
            - Followed by high dose protocol: biweekly 10 mg/kg up to three months postop, then monthly for months four through six. Then the dose drops to 5 mg/kg monthly thereafter.
            - Low dose protocol: monthly 10 mg/kg for month two and three. Followed by 5 mg /kg monthly thereafter.
    - BENEFIT study: Belatacept versus cyclosporine patients had higher PTLD (1.5% versus 0.4%) and

higher PML in EBV negative and now is C/I in that population.

- Long term shows higher early ACR (17%) versus Cys (7%) but better renal function in one year (GFR 63 ml / min / 1.73 m^2 versus 36.6 ml / min / 1.73 m^2). Late ACR rejection rates were the same.

Prefix	Target		Source		Suffix
Variable	-viI	viral	-u-	human	-mab (monoclonal Ab)
	I(c)	bacterial	-0-	mouse	
	-li(m)	immune	-a-	rat	-cept (fusion protein)
	-le(s)	infectious lesions	-e-	hamster	
	-ci(r)	cardiovascular	-i-	primate	
	-co(l)	colonic tumor	-xi-	chimeric	
	-me(l)	melanoma	-zu-	human-ized	

Thymoglobulin

Rabbits immunized from thymocytes retrieved from pediatric thymus glands, hence referred to as rATG (rabbit anti-Thymocyte globulin).
ATGAM is equine-derived ATG, used if rabbit Abs develops.
r-ARG is better than ATGAM (has improved tolerance and efficacy).
Dose is 1.5 mg/kg range; total for patient is 4–7 mg/kg, dependent on risk factors.
For example, African American, young, and high PRA patients would need a higher dose versus and older patient zero PRA, Caucasian.
Pretreatment requires giving Benadryl (50 mg), Methylprednisone, thirty minutes before thymo. Tylenol given before thymo and four hours after.
Peripheral administration is associated with thrombophlebitis, but new specific peripheral formulations allow this.

Extended half-life after repeated administration.

Large Number of Target Antigens:

- Binds to T cell → dose dependent depletion.
- Binds B cells.
- Binds macrophages.
    - Weak binding of PLTs, erythroocytes and neutrophils.
- APC: CD3 / TCR / CD38 / 40.
- Adhesion: CD11a and CD44.
- T cell specific: CD 4 / 8 / 45.
- MHC
- Cytokine receptors

- **Results In:**
    - Lymphocyte depletion dose dependent in the spleen and lymph nodes.
    - Long-term anergy and immunomodulation.
    - Altered B cell function → B-cell apoptosis, decreased B-cell proliferation, and inhibition of B-cell lymphoma.

Thymoglobulin and B Cells:

- Does not activate B cells.
- Does not cause their differentiation.
- Induces apoptosis of naïve / memory and active B cells / plasma cells.
- Inhibits EBV transformed lymphoblastoid B cells and Burritt's lymphomas.

Thymoglobulin and T Cells:

- Apoptosis: only affects activated T cells but not resting T cells. Leads to prolonged lymphopenia.
- Changes surface protein and hence decreases costimulatory signals and leads to anergy.
- Downmodulation of adhesion molecules and inflammatory molecules and results in decreased DGF / ischemia reperfusion injury.
- Inversion of CD4 (less): CD8 (more) after T-cell repopulation compared to pretransplant levels by twenty-four months—significance is unclear.

Use allows for delayed CNI initiation.

Also had lower subsequent acute rejections.

Most common complication was thrombocytopenia (half doses given for plt count 50,000–75,000 cells / ml).

Target an absolute lymphocyte count of 0.1%.

Maintenance Immunosuppression

Calcineurin Inhibitors (CNI):

- **FK (506), Also Known As Tacrolimus:** Streptomyces tsukubaensis, 1984 discovery in Japan, FDA approved 1994.
  - Ten to one hundred times in vitro activity of Cys.
  - $T_{1/2}$ = 8.5 hours.
  - Hepatic metabolized and excreted in bile, highest bioavailability in fasting and lower in postprandial.
  - Interaction with cytochrome inhibitors can affect its metabolism. Pediatric patients and African Americans may take longer to reach therapeutic levels; in fact sometimes ketoconazole is used as an agent to achieve therapeutic levels of tacrolimus without using high doses.
  - Available in PO, IV and SL form (SL is half the dose of PO form).
  - Major SE include tremors and neuro-related changes. It is also associated with new-onset diabetes mellitus (NODM).
  - Can increase mycophenolic acid exposure versus cyclosporine and mycophenolate exposure. In some circumstances switching to cyclosporine from tacrolimus is thought to lower mycophenolate acid exposure and immunosuppression—switch done in BK nephropathy.
- **Cyclosporine (Cys):** cyclic undecapeptide, FDA approved in 1983, discovered in 1973 in southern Norway from the fungus Beauveria nivea.
  - Prodrugs that are bound to immunophilins, for example, cyclophilin (Cys) or FK-BP 12 (Tacrolimus), block the phosphatase action of calcineurin, which

stops the T cell progressing from G0 to G1 phases by stopping IL-2 production.
- Cyclosporine is dependent on entero-hepatic recirculation; therefore patients with biliary disease or drains will have lower levels and be at risk of rejection.
- Sandimmune drug formulation is bile dependent absorption, versus Neoral is not.
- Adverse SE include gingival hyperplasia, hirsutism. It is also thought to result in lower graft GFR versus tacrolimus.
- Neurotoxicity higher with tacrolimus (range from tremor → seizures → coma).
    - Posterior reversible encephalopathy syndrome (PRES): headache, confusion, and visual loss.
        - Believed to be related to peak levels of tacrolimus that cross the blood brain barrier.
        - Marked by edema on MRI.
        - Improves with discontinuation. Rarely visual changes may remain.

- **Envarsus XR and Astagraf XR:** extended release tacrolimus, new formulation in the market that is supposed to avoid the S/E associated with the cyclic peaks and trough of BID tacrolimus (i.e., tremors and neurologic SE).
    - It is a once daily dose—easier compliance-wise. Dose is two-thirds of the combined dose of the bid tacrolimus (i.e., tacrolimus of three-thirds equals Envarsus four mg daily).
- Side effects of CNI:
    - Nephrotoxicity:
        - Decreased filtration: renal vasoconstriction that is dose related, especially afferent arteriole. May lead to delayed graft function. Some studies have looked into substituting CNI with belatacept for kidneys with high suspicion of DGF to bridge that early phase without straining the kidney with a

vasoconstrictive agent like a CNI. Also some studies have used low dose dopamine to encourage urine output in recipients immediately postop.
    - Interstitial fibrosis: resulting from the long term CNI use, which results in TGF-β.
    - TMA: thrombotic microangiopathy has similar pathology to TTP.
    - Hyperkalemia.

mTOR:

- Sirolimus, aka rapamycin: Streptomyces hygroscopicus, macrocyclic lactone (antibiotic), inhibits T-cell response to IL-2, FDA approved in 1999. Everolimus: has shorter half-life.
  - Prodrug binds FKBP12 at different site to CNIs, binds mTOR protein, and inhibits mTORC1 complex and inhibits progression from G1 → S phase.
  - Is not nephrotoxic alone but can potentiate CNI nephrotoxicity when used together but leads to delayed wound healing by decreasing fibroblast responsiveness. It is also associated with higher lymphoceles, proteinuria, diabetes.
  - Anti-tumor property especially SCC (TUMORAPA study), Kaposi, PTLD.
  - Also it inhibits the effects of steroids on monocytes and dendritic cells.
  - Other adverse effects:
    - Proteinuria: It should not be used if a patient already has proteinuria, and it should be checked on patients on it as de novo proteinuria can occur.
    - Localized limb angioedema: due to impaired lymphangiogenesis. Couse of ACE inhibitors may be a risk.
    - Pneumonia: Often necessitating prophylactic Bactrim for a year.

Antimetabolites:

Purine synthesis is either de novo pathway or salvage pathway. *T/B cell proliferation is dependent on de novo pathway and lacks the salvage pathway.* Other cell types can undergo salvage pathway.

- **MMF (Mycophenolate Mofetil), Also Known as CellCept:** 1995
- **Mycophenolate sodium (Myfortic):** 2004
  - Metabolite mycophenolate acid inhibits de novo pathway of purine biosynthesis, reversible selective, competitive inosine monophosphate dehydrogenase inhibitor (IMPDH). IMPDH catalyzed the inosine monophosphate → guanine monophosphate. With the lack of purine nucleotides, lymphocyte population is inhibited. It is more selective to lymphocytes versus azathioprine.
    - CellCept dose: early 1 g BID, later dose dropped to 500 mg BID. Can be given IV (in D5W).
    - Myfortic: given at 720 mg BID. Has fewer GI side effects, as it's enteric coated.
    - MMF had one-half of azathioprine rejection rates. But also lowers rate of late rejection.
    - Cyclosporine decreases the MMF absorption by decreasing its enterohepatic circulation.
    - SE: generally includes GI upset, although less with Myfortic, and bone marrow suppression.
- **Azathioprine:**
  - Blocks de novo purine synthesis and T cell costimulation signal.
    - 6-thio-GTP metabolite blocks T cell DNA replication and CD 28 (signal two pathway).
    - Not used with the advent of MMF.

Corticosteroids:

- **Prednisone / Methylpred:** Prodrugs broken to prednisolone by liver. Binds to Corticosteroid binding globulin, enters cell via diffusion or endocytosis. Binds cytosolic GR (glucocorticoid receptor), translocates across the nucleus and binds GRE (glucocorticoid receptor elements) of various genes and modulates their transcription:

- Downregulates APC (by down regulating IL-1/IL-6).
- Inhibits cytokine synthesis: affects wound healing too.
- Depletes circulating T cells:
  - Independent of cytokine pathways.
  - Also acts to decrease PKC-calcium pathways.
  - NFAT block.
  - Blockade AP1 (IL-2 promoter).
  - mRNASE of IL-2 gene.
- Adverse effect:
  - Cushingoid changes
  - Adrenal insufficiency
  - Avascular necrosis
  - Osteoporosis
  - Hyperglycemia
  - Cataracts
  - CVA / CAD
- Early steroid withdrawal:
  - Within four to five days of induction with rapid taper.
  - Benefit must outweigh the risk of rejection, therefore not done in high PRA prior transplants.

Organ Procurements

Organ Preservation Fluids

1849—First published.
1953—Hypothermic kidney and limbs.
1979—(UW) University Wisconsin, aka Belzer.
1981—HTK (histidine-tryptophan-ketoglutarate)—initial use was as cardioplegic solution.

Preservation Fluids Goal:

Prevents Cell Swelling and Tissue Edema:

- Hydroxyethyl starch, lactobionate, mannitol, raffinose, tryptophan.

Maintain Intracellular PH:

- Histidine.

Allows Substrate for ATP Generation:

- Adenosine, ketoglutarate, L-arginine.

Free Radical Injury Protection:

- Glutathione, allopurinol, N-AC.

Ischemia-Reperfusion Physiology:

- Mitochondrial dysfunction and loss of ATP production →dysfunctional Na/K ATPase and Ca+ channels → influx of Na+ cell swelling, Ca+ influx and loss of signaling

pathway and free radical production → cell DNA and cellular damage.
- Hypothermia is used in both static and pulsatile preservation (extracorporeal perfusion at two to eight degrees Celsius temperature) to limit this injury.

Most Commonly Used Preservation Fluids Are:
- **UW** (Na+ / High K+ / raffinose / lactobionate / hydroxyethyl starch / glutathione / adenosine).
- **HTK** (In addition to H/T/K, also has mannitol and K+ / Na+).

Comparison Properties:
- UW (very high K+)—organs, especially the liver, need to be flushed well before implantation, as to avoid potentially lethal hyperkalemia
- HTK is less viscous than UW—potential better microvasculature penetration.
- HTK is cheaper per liter than UW. Three to six liters used during procurements.
- HTK has controversial use with majority showing it inferior to UW in liver / kidney / pancreas, and even more prominent in ECD or organs with increased cold ischemia time (less than twenty-four hours).
- Hard to pinpoint completely on fluid type as procurement practices and IS have changed with time.
- During the cooling process and storage, when cells cool, the ATP utilization falls, which causes the intracellular sodium level to rise, resulting in lethal cell swelling, and that is why a lot of our preservative fluids use saccharides and large anions to mitigate that effect. Hence mannitol is used in the Euro-Collins, Belzer' MPS, HTK, Celsior and custodial-N fluids

Kidneys Preserved on Pumps:
- Decreased DGF. Same one / three year graft survival.

- Increased interest in use with DCD and ECD kidneys to lower discard rate. (Rate of ECD kidneys discarded that were pumped was 30% versus 44% unpumped).
- Optimal pump parameters:
  - Kidney flow ≥ 100 ml/min.
  - Kidney renovascular resistance index (RI) < 0.4.
  - Systolic Perfusion pressure < 50 mmHg.
- 11/89 kidneys meeting poor perfusion RI > 0.4 mmHg / flow 80 ml/min had good kidney function after transplantation after being pumped.

Livers Preserved on Pumps:

- First study that studied forty organs (twenty on pump versus standard preservation).
- Livers exclusion criteria: DCD, donor > sixty-five years, > 25% steatosis, MELD > 35.
- Organs pumped for three to seven hours with total CIT < twelve hours.
- Livers on the pump:
  - Less early allograft dysfunction (5% versus 25%).
  - Shorter LOS (ten versus fifteen days).
  - NO PNF or vascular complications.
  - Two had biliary complications.

Abdominal Organ Procurement

Prior to surgery:

- ABO compatible.
- Medical / surgical history.
- Serology.
- Latest labs / imaging.
- OR equipment.
- Respectful.

Operation:

- **Principles:**
  - Preservation of perfusion until aortic clamp.
  - Rapid cooling: Topical and infusion.
  - Exsanguination.
  - Perfusion of organs: preserve vascular length when possible.
- **Surgery**:
  - Confirm patient.
  - Anesthesiologist: heparin / muscle relaxant, fluid expectations.
  - Nursing / surgical tech: cautery times two, two to three suctions, sternal saw / Lebsche knife.
  - Teams: time of clamping.
  - Inspect organs r/o cancer. Mobilize left lobe.
  - Exposure of hepatic vessels in the warm versus cold.
  - Catell-Braach—Kocher.
  - Inferior Mesenteric Vein (IMV) cannulation.
  - Encircle aorta above bifurcation—beware of lumbar branches / Inferior Mesenteric Artery (IMA) / low accessory renal arteries.
  - Portal triad dissection—dissect common bile duct (CBD). Ligate distally and cut—flush gall bladder.

- Open lesser sac—LHA accessory be aware.
- Supra celiac—clamp.
- Heparinization.

Extra Steps for Pancreas Recovery:

- En-bloc resection with liver versus sequential with the liver.
- Optional: Betadyne and or amphotericin in duodenum.
- Divide short gastrics.
- Mobilization of spleen / pancreas.
- Division of duodenum distal to the pylorus.
- Division of D3 at the SMA after the clamp.

- **Pediatric Donors:**
  - Assume accessory arteries—clear at back table.
  - PV taken back to SMV / SV.
  - Thoracic organs used as the conduits.
  - Take iliac vessels.
  - Notify abnormal changes to recipient surgeon and estimated return time.

Brain-Dead Donors

Confirmatory Tests:

- Neurological exam—brain stem reflexes.
- EEG.
- Apnea test, ten minutes lead to CO_2 rise of greater than sixty or twenty-four above baseline with no respiratory effort.
- Nuclear imaging.
- Cerebral angiography.

Exclusion Criteria:

- Under sedation / hypothermia.

Physiologic Changes:

- **Hemodynamic Effects:**
  - **Autonomic Storm:** tachycardia, HTN, increased SVR—short lived.
    - Anaerobic metabolic, glycogen depletion, lactate accumulation. **Tx: nitroprusside / esmolol gtt.**
  - **Loss of Sympathetic Tone:** edema, hypotension, and functional hypovolemia. Tx: dopamine / NE gtt, in low cardiac output dobutamine may be used.
  - Myocardial ischemia.

- **Temperature Control:**
  - Hypothalamic injury.

- H**ormonal / Endocrine Instability:**
  - Hypothyroidism / low ACTH, GH, low cortisol, low ADH—diabetes insipidus. Tx: Vasopressin + D5, steroids, Insulin gtt, T4 infusion.
- **Pulmonary Injury:**

    - ARDS occurs in 15–20% of BD patients.
    - Systemic hypoxemia.
- **DIC:**
    - High plasminogen activator.
- **Electrolyte Abnormalities:**
    - Hypernatremia—worst outcome on liver transplant.

Unusual Circumstances:

- Directed donation.
- Crashing donor.
- Compassionate request.
- Rerunning of match list if initial data was incorrect.
- Kidney will follow life-saving organ (heart → liver → pancreas).

Donor Cancer:

- CNS versus non-CNS:
    - CNS
        - GBM / medulloblastomas are the only CNS considered high risk.
            - Shunts—high risk.
    - Non-CNS:
        - Skin except melanoma: considered OK.
        - Staging and years from cancer (low stage cancer, two to five years cancer free, dependent on cancer type—is considered low risk).
            - Below is a useful table of donor cancer risk.

Donor Infection:

- Localized versus systemic.
- Intra-abdominal contamination.
- Meningitis:
    - Bacterial with offending bug identified is usable.
    - Viral—risky.

Transmission Risk from Donor to Recipient	Type of Malignancy
Minimal (<0.1% transmission risk)	Non Melanoma Skin cancer
	In situ Cervical / Vocal cord cancer
	Thyroid: Solitary Papillary ≤0.5cm Minimally invasive Follicular carcinoma ≤ 1cm
	Renal Cell carcinoma: Solitary resected ≤1cm well differentiated Fuhrman 1-2)
Low risk (0.1-1% transmission risk)	Renal Cell carcinoma: Solitary resected >1cm ≤2.5cm well differentiated Fuhrman 1-2)
	CNS tumor: Low grade (WHO grade 1/2) CNS primary teratoma
	Thyroid: Solitary Papillary 0.5cm- 2cm Minimally invasive Follicular carcinoma 1cm -2cm
	Non-CNS treated malignancy ≥5 years with 99% cure probability
Intermediate risk (1-10% transmission risk)	Breast cancer: In-Situ
	Colon Cancer: In-Situ
	Renal Cell carcinoma: Solitary resected T1b (4cm-7cm) well differentiated Fuhrman 1-2)
	Non-CNS treated malignancy ≥5 years with 90-99% cure probability
High risk (>10% transmission risk)	Malignant melanoma (active or history of)
	Breast cancer: >stage 0
	Colon Cancer: > stage 0
	CNS tumor: Grade (WHO grade 3/4) Any CNS tumor needing shunting / surgical resection/ irradiation or with extra CNS metastasis
	Leukemia / Lymphoma (active or history of)
	Metastatic Carcinoma
	Sarcoma
	Lung Cancer (Stages I-IV)
	Renal Cell carcinoma: >7cm or (Stage II-IV)
	Small cell/ neuroendocrine Carcinoma at any site (active or history of)
	Active cancer not listed above
	Non-CNS treated malignancy with insufficient follow up period or considerd incurable or with <90% sure rate.

Figure 1. Table from Donor-Transmitted Malignancies in Organ Transplantation: Assessment of Clinical Risk. *American Journal of Transplantation* 2011; 11: 1140–1147.

Controlled Donation after Cardiac Death

- Irreversible circulatory arrest.
- Increasing use.
- Initial data when comparing liver DCD organs versus DBD—outcomes looked worse especially at five years. However, when low risk DCD (CIT less than ten, WIT less than fifteen minutes, donor age less than forty-five) are looked at, the outcomes were the same as DBD organs.

Meds Used:

- Most allow use of heparin prior to removal of support unless it is going to hasten death.
- Morphine—depends on patients' treating team.
- Phentolamine—depends on center.
- Two- to five-minute waiting period to make sure autoresuscitation does not occur.
- Declaration of death.
- Mannitol and Lasix is also used.

Technique:

- **Modified Pittsburgh Super Rapid Technique:**
  - Rapid laparotomy: Two Kochers, either side of umbilicus.
  - Distal aortic cannulation—use umbilical tape to secure flush but use Kelly for distal occlusion to flush—start flush immediately.
  - Flush and ice cooling.
  - Sternal split, thoracic aortic lamping.
  - Vent prior to engorgement—if concern, may be able to vent prior to cross clamp.

    - Flush biliary tree.
    - Portal flush in situ or back table.

- Premortem cannulation (arterial / venous used for flushing) needs specific consent, may be used if there is concern that there will be delay to moving to the OR.

WIT / CIT Times Acceptable for Organs:

- Liver: WIT less than twenty to thirty minutes, CIT less than eight to ten hours.
- Kidney: WIT less than forty to sixty minutes, CIT less than twenty-four hours.
- Pancreas: WIT less than forty-five to sixty minutes, CIT less than eighteen hours.
-
- Use of Ex Vivo pumps for DCD kidneys has improved DGF rates.
- However, some reports have associated DCD liver with increasing ischemic cholangiopathy.

In one study from Johns Hopkins comparing the use of DCD kidneys from the elderly more than fifty years old, donor versus not, showed there was an increased mortality risk in the first months postop: 1.3% versus 0.5% (nonacceptors). But there is an exponential almost patient survival the further out at one to five years, for those acceptors versus those nontransplanted. Ultimately it was associated with a 41% risk of decreased mortality.

Dialysis Access

Arterio-Venous Fistula

Sixty percent of ESRD patients are on hemodialysis (HD).

Cost > 200 million a year.

Vascular access is associated with 25% of all ESRD-related inpatient admissions.

Arterio-Venous fistula (AVF) is preferred to grafts in diabetics and nondiabetics. Followed by AV grafts, followed by tunneled catheters.

Catheters Tunneled—intermediate solution.

Also the first type of access has an implication on AVF failure rate; therefore, early referral is essential.

- Both in the US / European studies, AVF with no prior CVC or temporary access had higher / better / longer access survival rates.
- PICC basilic vein is associated with rates of central venous stenosis or thrombosis estimated up to 85%.

DOQI Guidelines: Aim for 65% of ESRD to have of AVF.

Principles for Placing AVF:

- Nondominant first.
- Distal first.
- Avoid diseased vessels.
- Easy to cannulate.
- Perfection in creation.
- Prophylactic antibiotic use, especially if graft is used.

- Do not r/o AVF because of age.
- CO_2 contrast imaging if needed.
- Always check for Allen's Test.

Order of Choice:

- Radial-cephalic, also known as Cimino: traditionally at wrist level, simple lower comps risk; however, low flow rate.
- Modified—below elbow level.
- Brachial-Cephalic: above antecubital fossa. Higher blood flow, easier cannulation, increased steal syndrome, and more complicated surgically.
- Transposed basilic vein brachiobasilic: move basilic vein from deep medial to the more superficial and lateral position. Extensive surgery performed in two stages most of the time.
- AV graft (PTFE) preferred to Dacron, etc. Also cadaveric grafts and bovine grafts are potential.
- CVC to allow time for fistulas to mature.

Preop Eval:

- CVD risk (CHF+ DM, PVD, CVA, CAD, HTN).
- Prior Access (pacemakers, CL, PICC, defibrillators)
- Trauma to UE / clavicles.
- Palpate RA, UA, BA Allen's test—if using radiocephalic.
- Cephalic vein assessment via tourniquet and palpating vein in forearm from wrist to antecubital fossa.
- Vein mapping may be helpful in those who are obese, intravenous drug abusers, or have had prior PICC lines.
- Preop venography is used to assess central vein patency in patients with history of arm swelling—carbon dioxide used a contrast agent.
- X-rays for IVDU to r/o FB.
- Preop DDAVP 0.3 µg/kg ASA 81 not held. Plavix is held five to seven days preop. Coumadin—not withheld.

Procedure:

- Local for radiocephalic and brachiocephalic with no transposition.
- Infraclavicular regional nerve blocks are preferred.
- Deltopectoral skin incisions will need additional local anesthetic with the regional infraclavicular block.
- Supraclavicular blocks were associated with SOB with phrenic nerve paresis.
- If the brachial artery appears smaller than expected, the patient most likely has a high brachial bifurcation. Deeper branch is often better.
- Arteriotomy greater than one cm is at higher risk of steal syndrome; too small, though, can lead to failure of maturation.
- Six-mm ePTFE, bovine carotid artery, bovine mesenteric vein, and polyurethane-urea (Vectra, BARD Peripheral Vascular, Inc., Tempe, Arizona) grafts also may be used.
- The venous anastomosis is performed first (when using ePTFE; however, if using a biologic graft, the arterial anastomosis is performed first), particularly if the graft has a premade flared end.

Alternatives in Difficult Access:

- The HeRO (Hemodialysis Reliable Outflow):
  - Standard ePTFE graft and a reinforced single lumen venous outflow catheter wired across stenosis to the right atrium.
  - The other end of the catheter is then tunneled laterally to the deltopectoral groove and attached to the standard ePTFE graft via a manufacturer-supplied alloy connector. The ePTFE graft is then tunneled like any other graft, and the opposite end is sewn to the brachial artery in the standard fashion.
  - Chronic warfarin anticoagulation should be considered strongly in all patients being dialyzed via a HeRO graft.

- Low volume access (radial or ulnar based). Low-flow state that might be operable even with central vein stenosis without significant arm selling.
- Leg access: paraplegics → use arms for mobility; women → scarring aesthetic.
    - Loop ePTFE thigh is used.
    - Autogenous femoral vein used best in thin legs. Saphenous superficial tunneling can be used but often is small < 5 mm and fails to mature.
    - The graft inflow from deep femoral or proximal superficial femoral artery and outflow is the SFJ (preferentially).

Complications:

- **Thrombosis:** if early is often a technical complication, late is related to venous intimal hyperplasia, Tx interventional plasty / stent / jump graft/ revision.
- **Venous HTN:** *arm swelling*, MCC occult venous drainage obstruction, especially previous lines or traumas to chest / neck.
- **Arterial steal:** Especially diabetics, as they have narrow lumen vessels. Check with Allen's Test. Higher risk in brachiocephalic versus radiocephalic.
- **High output cardiac failure**: CHF.
- **Neuropathy**: trauma versus ischemia related.
- **Infection:** limb and life threatening especially in graft. Lower risk in fistulas. Requires emergent surgical management.
- **Aneurysm:** pseudo versus true.

Complications of Vascular Access:

Two-thirds of all accesses will fail at some point.
For a fistula to be used for dialysis in the United States, the flow needs to be at least 350 ml/min.

Risk of primary fistula failure was 34% lower when the fistulae were created by surgeons that had exceeded twenty-five fistulas during their training.

Presentation of Inflow Problems:

- Not matured fistula despite time (six weeks considered adequate).
  - Hard to cannulate.
  - Collapsing arterial inflow.
- Inflow of the fistula is decreasing steadily.
- Lack of bruit and thrill indicates thrombosis.
- A weak thrill or bruit suggests inflow problems.

Presentation Outflow Problems:

- High venous pressures.
- Aneurysmal dilatation.
- Excessive bleed after decannulation.
- Pulsatility in a fistula generally indicates an outflow venous problem.

Image:

- US / CTA / Fistulogram.

Thrombosis:

- Angiographic mechanical thrombectomy.

Maturation:

- **Rule of Sixes:**
  - Within *six weeks* of creation.
    - 600 cc of blood / min.
    - 6 mm deep—to cannulate.
    - 6 mm in diameter.
    - 6 cm of vein length to cannulate.
- Studies have shown that the best fistula maturation rates occur when the venous outflow is greater than or equal to 2.5 mm and the arterial inflow is greater than or equal to 2 mm.

Physiology:

- Shunting—avoiding capillaries due to lower resistance through vein.
- Venous and arterial dilatation due to increased CO (ten to twenty fold in exercise).

RF Failed Maturation Risk Factors:

- Female
- Radiocephalic
- Small veins
- Diabetes
- Obesity

Complications:

- **Tortuous + extravasation:** Option to resect excess fistula length and perform end-to-end anastomosis.
- **Deep and unable to cannulate due to obesity:** transpose fistula more superficially.
- **Venous Neointimal Hyperplasia (stenosis):** angioplasty
  - Six month patency is 50% if it occurs—no long-term viable treatment.
  - Covered stents still: 50% patency at one year best.
- **Fistula infections:**
  - Treated with antibiotics—even PO Staph MC organism.
- **Graft infections:** Need surgery: resect entire graft, repair vessels, tunneled cath. Same-time reconstruction is not recommended.
- **Accessory veins** (side branches) mainly in forearm AVF but should always rule a central or downstream stenosis, which should be treated first.
  - One study found that preoperatively detected accessory veins with a diameter > 70% of the cephalic vein diameter had a high risk of radiocephalic nonmaturation.

- Treatment:
  - Percutaneous ligation blind double stitch remains for ten days.
  - Surgical ligation (can be spasmodic and might need a guidewire across to aid in localization).
  - Coil embolization (coil slightly larger than vein so it doesn't migrate).
- **Thrombosis:** if it occurs early , it is often a technical complication, late occurrence is often related to venous intimal hyperplasia, Tx interventional plasty / stent / jump graft/ revision.
- **Venous HTN:** *arm swelling*, MCC occult venous drainage obstruction, especially previous lines or traumas to chest / neck.
- **Arterial steal:**
  - Significant steal occurs less than 15% of the time, brachial artery–based accesses presenting the highest risk.
  - Especially diabetics as they have narrow lumen vessels.
  - Check with Allen's Test.
  - Loss of a palpable distal pulse at the time of fistula creation indicates that a significant steal syndrome could develop.
  - Manual compression of the fistula should result in restoration of the distal pulse.
  - Ligation, plication, banding, proximalization of the arterial inflow, and the distal revascularization with internal ligation (DRIL) procedure.
- **High-output cardiac failure**: CHF.
- **Neuropathy**: trauma versus ischemia related, if associated with steal syndrome, may need surgical revision; however if in cutaneous distribution over incision site, may be recoverable with time.
- **Aneurysm:** pseudo versus true.

Arterial-Venous Grafts

Imminent HD needed; cannot wait for maturation.
Poor superficial vein quality for AVF.
Larger anatomic target potentials.

Conduits used include PTFE, bovine carotid artery, bovine mesenteric vein, and human umbilical vein.
PTFE structural and coating advances to improve longevity.

Biologic Grafts:

- Saphenous vein transposition versus PTFE:
  - There were significantly more infectious complications with the PTFE over the vein but more venous anastomotic stenosis and slightly more aneurysms in the preserved vein over the PTFE graft but similar patency rates versus inferior vein patency on some studies.
- Cadaveric treated vein donors have antigenicity risk that can affect future transplants.
- Mandil graft not used.
- Bovine carotid graft in one study had better primary patency and longevity versus ePTFE but same secondary patency rates.
- Bovine ureteric grafts: no clear advantage to their use.

Synthetic Grafts:

- Dacron has less durability with the multiple punctures versus PTFE.
- Size, construction, layering variations to PTFE that is operator choice.
- Derivatives of PTFE that can be used immediately include polyurethane or multilayered PTFE, as it has an auto sealant property.

Surgery:

Silva et al. looked at the preoperative assessment including ultrasound interrogation for a noninvasive assessment of the vasculature and found that a feeding arterial lumen of 2.0 mm or more and a draining vein diameter of 4.0 mm or more were associated with better success in dialysis graft placement.

The use of arterial clamps on the graft while performing graft placement is associated with a lower graft survival rate.

The use of the axillary vein for the venous outflow is associated with better outcomes.

The use of the brachial artery over the radial artery with an anastomotic angle of less than ninety degrees is also associated with a better graft survival rate.

This incorporation can prevent perigraft fluid accumulation or hematoma despite repetitive puncture; therefore delay first cannulation of a graft for at least two weeks unless a compelling reason to use the device sooner arises.

Disadvantage:

Lower patency versus AVF (500 versus 1500 median days), 9% versus 51% average five year patency rate.

Higher intervention rate—cost.

Higher incidence of steal syndrome on HD.

Peritoneal Dialysis

Hyperosmolar dialysate used to remove toxins across peritoneal membrane.
Less expensive.
Three components of membrane:

- Mesothelial: Not involved
- Interstitium: not involved
- Capillary wall:
    - Pore system—that allows the dialysis solute's movement across a concentration gradient.
        - Which leads to DM eventually.
            - Most of the water transfers through ultrapores, aka aquaporins.

Membrane failure factors:

- Adhesions—less surface area (SA)
- Inflammation—high (SA).
- Hernias.
- Patient capable of self-care / motivation / lifestyle.

Catheter:

- Double cuff
    - First cuff rests at the rectus sheath, second at subcutaneous.

Can be done:

- Open versus laparoscopic versus percutaneous.

General principles:

- Single dose antibiotics sixty minutes before surgery to decrease infection.

- Clearly placed in true pelvis.
- Paramedian placement with downward facing exit.

Complications:

- Peritonitis 0.25-0.5 episode / patient / year.
    - S. Aureus MC organism.
    - Tx: intraperitoneal abs.
    - Remove the catheter.
    - Look at other potential causes (e.g., diverticulitis).
- Surgical site infection:
    - Daily cleaning
    - Gentamicin topical treatment
- Catheter migration:
    - Lateral / AP views with X-ray.
    - Use catheters with weighted tips / suturing (PD pexy).
- Catheters occlusion:
    - Fibrin declot / omentectomy
- Bleeding.
- Catheter leak.

Postop Care:

- Dressed for seven to ten days.
- Antiseptic cleaning of exit site qday—keeping catheter immobile.
- Topical antimicrobials.

Kidney Transplant

Pre–Kidney Transplant Evaluation

Aim:

- Risk stratification.
- Inform patient of the process.
- Formulate plans and strategies with the patient.
- Loop communication to referring physician.

Indications for Kidney Txp (transplant):

- ESRD (end-stage renal disease) on PD (peritoneal dialysis) or HD (hemodialysis) or preemptive (not on dialysis yet) with GFR < twenty cc/min.

Evaluations:

- **Etiology** of their ESRD +/– Bx (renal biopsy may be needed).
    - Do they need also a pancreas transplant?
        - Simultaneous pancreas and kidney versus pancreas after kidney versus sequential living kidney followed by pancreas (see pre–pancreas transplant eval chapter).
- **Dialysis** type / duration / complications on dialysis (e.g., access / hypotension / clotting / compliance)—indicator of hypercoagulability, need for access prior to surgery / points for wait list.
- **Urologic** evaluation—stones / malignancy / surgeries. Quantify how much urine they make baseline; this can guide you on how well a graft is functioning posttransplant.

- **Weight** changes minus dry weight equals weight after dialysis (to evaluate volume status posttransplant) / cachexia / obesity.
- **Hospitalizations**: Past medical history (PMHx), surgical Hx, social Hx, anesthesia Hx.
- **Cardiac evals** (see preop cardiac evaluation chapter).
- **Functional** status—Karnofsky eval (fifty to sixty average score of those on chronic HD) reflects level of independence.
- **Cancer screening**.
- **Operative plan:** Donor selection for ECD (extended criteria donor) versus SCD (standard criteria donor): see next chapter. Site (left / right). Retroperitoneal versus intraabdominal.

Physical Exam:

- Remember **femoral pulse exam** character and strength, especially important in diabetics as they may have peripheral vascular disease.
- **Access:** is it currently functional? Previous fistulas or lines used (any in the groin) will affect kidney transplant site.
- **Previous scars and surgeries**: operative plan.

Labs:

- **Basic workup:** CBC, CMP, coags, HLA / PRA, typing, albumin, serologies (CMV / EBV / Hep C, Hep B, HIV), CXR.
- **Hypercoagulable workup**: Factor V, prothrombin G20201A, lupus, cardiolipin, antiphospholipid, protein c/s, antithrombin, homocysteine.
- **Autoimmune activity**: lupus (dsDNA, C3, CH50) Wegener's (ANCA), Goodpasture's (anti-GBM).

Social work evaluation:

- Compliance.
- Social support.
- Financial support.

Preoperative Cardiac Evaluation and Management

Leading cause of postop mortality in kidney transplant (30%, highest within first month of transplant).
Transplant does improve risk of cardiovascular disease versus dialysis.

Evaluation:
Thorough history and exam.
Twelve lead EKG (25% will worsen at a 7.5 year follow-up), (Pathologic Q waves were most associated with an abnormal MPS).
ECHO (preferred to be done when patient has reached dry weight).
Referral to *assigned* cardiologist who clears transplant patients.

High-risk patients (based on Lisbon report) should get cardiac stress test (Dobutamine stress ECHO [DSE] or Myocardial perfusion scan [MPS] or exercise treadmill test), and repeated annually while on wait list:

- Diabetic.
- Prior ischemic heart disease.
- ≥ two traditional cardiac risk factors.
- Peripheral arterial disease.
- LVEF ≤ 40%.
- > Sixty years.
- > One year on dialysis.
- Smoking, HTN, HLD.

Between 3% and 9.5% of pretransplant cardiac evaluated patients end up requiring PCI / revascularization (bypass).

DSE and MPS are very imperfect at identifying one or more CAD with ≥ 70% stenosis, in ESRD patients.
Although they have similar sensitivity 0.79 versus 0.74, respectively, and specificity of 0.89 versus 0.79, respectively, some studies suggested improved DSE over MPS P = 0.02.
Associations with coronary stenoses and subsequent CAD events are inconsistent. This may be because plaque instability (erosion or rupture) is a more important factor in major adverse cardiac events (MACE) versus actually stenotic sites.
(CARP and DECREASE-V trial). There is, however, a lack of evidence for the PCI over medical therapy in asymptomatic patients with CAD except in cases of 3-vessel CAD.

Symptomatic patients who need revascularization:

- CABG: is recommended over PCI for multivessel CAD and diabetic patients, especially if internal mammary graft was used.
- Indicated:
  - > 50% left main stenosis.
  - > 70% three major vessels.
  - > 70% in proximal LAD + one other major vessel.
- Timing of transplantation after intervention:
  - > Twelve month for patients with drug eluting stents.
  - > Three months for bare metal stents (usually after one month the stent has full endothelial coverage); six months is when restenosis may occur.
  - > One month for balloon angioplasty.

Prognosis: postrevascularization (CABG or PCI) ESRD patients have worse mortality compared to the general population (28% five-year survival versus 80–90% five-year survival, respectively)

Other imaging:
Noncontrast Cardiac CT:

Significantly improve cardiovascular risk prediction in patients with ESRD, through the quantification of coronary artery calcification (CAC).

Elevated scores of Agatston score median of 595 were associated with CAD. No strong evidence to suggest its validity in ESRD patients as the calcifications in them may be in tunica media versus intimal plaque atherosclerosis.

Cardiac troponin:

Elevated in ESRD, but levels ≥ 0.10 ng/ml were prognostic (50%–60% associated with higher two- to three-year cardiac events. Its role in guiding further workup is unclear.

Coronary angiography:

Reserved to abnormal noninvasive testing in order to reduce risks and associated costs.

Kidney Deceased Donor Selection

SCD (standard criteria donors)—kidneys from donors aged ten to thirty-nine, terminal Scr < 1.5, no HTN and no CVA.

ECD (extended criteria donor) formulated in Crystal City, Virginia, in 2001.
Donors with RF (risk factors) that are associated with a 70% increased risk of graft failure at one year versus SCD.
Translates to an 83% versus 90% graft survival at one year.

- ECD:
  - Donor > sixty years regardless of other factors.
  - Donor fifty to fifty-nine years and with two of the following:
    - HTN / CVA / serum creatinine (creat) > 1.5

RR graft failure (1.74–2.69)—highest for > sixty in age followed by death from CVA then creat > 1.5.

Kidney Grades based on deceased donor scoring (DDS) A, B, C, or D:

- ECD kidneys by definition were either grade C or D.
- Grade C:
  - Thirty percent had good GFR (GFR forty to sixty) at one year.
  - Twenty percent had poor (< 20 GFR) kidney function at one year.
- Grade D:
  - Twenty percent had good function GFR at one year.
  - Thirty percent had poor (GFR < 20) kidney function at one year.

Machine preservation (pump) can help evaluate further kidney function:

- Machine preservation in Europe has reduced DGF (delayed graft function) and primary nonfunction and improved graft survival at one year (94% versus 90%).
  - It is used if DDS is > twenty (i.e., ECD).
    - If RI (resistive index) ≥ 0.5, the kidney is discarded.

Maryland Aggregate Pathology Index (MAPI) score:
This is a preimplantation kidney biopsy score that has helped further risk stratify ECD kidneys.
Scores based on:

- Global glomerulosclerosis > 15% (two points).
- Arterial wall to lumen ratio (i.e., measure of vascular sclerosis) > 0.5 (two points).
- Arteriolar hyalinosis (four points).
- Parenchymal fibrosis and tubular atrophy involving at least ten tubules (three points).
- Periglomerular fibrosis, affecting Bowman's capsule (four points).

Low score (zero to seven)—had 95% five-year graft survival (despite organs labeled as ECD). Intermediate score (eight to eleven)—had 63% five-year graft survival). High score (twelve to fifteen)—had worst five-year graft survival (53%).

Recipient scoring system factors:

- Age, DM, angina, time on dialysis.

It is most beneficial to match the DDS and recipient scoring system.

Kidney Donor Risk Index: Estimate of graft longevity based on a multivariable analysis of risk factors for graft loss after deceased donor kidney transplant. The identifying factors included HLA match, CIT, en bloc, and dual kidney (aka two-for-one adult) coefficients + the ten KDPI factors listed below.

KDPI (kidney donor profile index): potential horsepower of kidney devoid of immunologic or candidate issues (i.e., the relative risk of graft failure compared to the median kidney from last year). KDPI > 85% needs a special consent by recipient (they are aware of the quality of the kidney). Pediatric transplants only allowed KDPI ≤ 35%, prioritization.

KDPI is based on ten factors:

- Age / ethnicity / HTN / DM / serum creatinine / HCV (ab) / weight / height / HTN / donor type (DCD or DBD).

It is imperative to note that KDPI does not take into account dual kidneys or en bloc kidneys; it is strictly for a single kidney. It is limited in that it does not estimate the KDRI on the DonorNet.

Estimated posttransplant survival (EPTS):

- Score based on:
  - Age / DM / prior Txp / years on HD.

Patients with the lowest 20% EPTS are matched to the lowest 20% KDPI = longevity matching.
Kidneys with KDPI > 20% are not matched this way.

New allocation system, aka KAS (kidney allocation system) also includes:

- Sensitization scoring through the PRA (panel-reactive antibodies = % of population to which a recipient would react):
  - Increase donor access for the highly sensitized recipients (i.e., the more sensitized a patient, the greater pull of organs they can have across regions):
    - Local cPRA 98%.
    - Regional cPRA 99%.
    - National cPRA 100%.

- Time of start of dialysis or when GFR < 20 ml/min.
- Kidney first goes with multiorgan, priority to life-saving organ (e.g., SLK before a SPK, etc.), (11% of kidneys).
- Screen blood group B patient for non-A1 kidney for possibly A2 kidney matching.

CDC Increased Risk Donors:

Donors with negative serologies or NAT (nucleic acid testing) but with high-risk behaviors that put them at risk for Hep B / Hep C or HIV:

- **MSM:** Men who had sex with another man in the last twelve months.
- Women who had sex with MSM behavior in the last twelve months.
- **IDU:** IV / IM / SC use of drugs in the last twelve months.
- **Prostitution:** Men or women doing this in exchange for money or drugs in the last twelve months.
- People who had sex with a person who had sex in exchange for money or drugs in the last twelve months.
- People having sex with people with known or suspected HIV / Hep B / Hep C in the last twelve months.
- **Birth:** A child eighteen months old born to a mother infected or who is at increased risk for HIV / Hep B / Hep C.
- A child who has been breastfed within the preceding twelve months by a mother who is infected or at increased risk for HIV.
- **Jail:** People who have been in lockup, jail, prison, or juvenile correctional facility for more than seventy-two consecutive hours in the preceding twelve months.
- **STD:** Donor with a recent diagnosis or treatment of syphilis, chlamydia, gonorrhea, or genital ulcers in the preceding twelve months.
- Donors who have started hemodialysis in the last twelve months are also considered at increased risk for Hep C.

Kidney–Living Donor Evaluation

Outcome:

Living donor superior to graft and patient survival in one to three years versus SCD kidney donors.

Rising unrelated living donors versus plateauing living related donor curve.

- May be partly due to national donor exchange programs for sensitized patients.

1950s: First living donor—Boston.

Aim:

- Safety.
- Minimal morbidity.
- Donor desire for good recipient outcome.

Risks on Donors:

No adverse risks on donor renal function, risks of hypertension or glomerular disease at ten to fifteen years post nephrectomy. Studied well, especially WWII veterans with unilateral nephrectomy study. Their risk of HTN and renal impairment is equivalent to the nondonors'.

Evaluation:

Evaluating team needs to be different from recipient team.

Donors evaluation, difficulties:

- Aging and increasing obesity population.

No gold standard available—based on institutional protocols.

Amsterdam Forum looked at RF:

- **HTN:** > 140 / 90 mmHg is a contraindication. Need ambulatory blood pressure monitoring to confirm if hypertensive. Those who are not SBP < 135 or DBP < 85, who are low risk (i.e., not AA), no evidence of end organ damage (microalbuminuria, no hypertrophy on echo), on single agent antihypertensive meds or low-dose combination antihypertensives. May be considered.
- **Obesity ≥ thirty-five BMI:** weight loss recommended first. Some centers' cutoff is a BMI thirty. Patients had a RR of ESRD three time if BMI was thirty to thirty-five and five times if BMI was thirty-five to forty.
- **Metabolic syndrome:** Male waist ≥ forty inches / female waist ≥ thirty-five inches + two from below:
    - HLD TG ≥ 150 mg/dl or on lipid lowering agent.
    - HDL ≤ 40 mg/dL.
    - SBP ≥ 135 mmHg.
    - DBP ≥ 85 mmHg.
    - Fasting blood glucose ≥ 100 mg/dL.
  - It is not a C/I in old donors but should be for young donors.
- **Age:** > Sixty-five—relative contraindication, center based.
- **DM:** Those with two times fasting glucose > 125 mg/dL or 7.0 mmol/L, OGTT > 200 mg/dL or 11.1 mmol/L are excluded.
  - FPG 100–125 will need OOGTT and HbA1C.
  - Donors with RF—first-degree relative with DM, Hx of gestational DM, > nine pounds birth weight or any metabolic syndrome like features or increase race group (Hispanic, Native American, Pacific Islander, and East Asian) will also need OGTT and HbA1C.
  - IFG (impaired fating glucose) (110–125 mg/dL) and IGT impaired glucose tolerance (140–199 mg/dL) are contraindicated if they carry any of the above RF or if IFG is in high range (110–125 mg/dL).
- **Urologic abnormalities**: Reflux disease is contraindication.

- **Microscopic hematuria (> three to five RBC/HPF):** Isolated event is not a contraindication; persistent events will need evaluation—urologic workup and renal biopsy even. Any concerns with that workup can make it a contraindication. Check sediment / casts.
- **Asymptomatic bacteriuria:** is common in females; pyuria is key determinant if treatment is needed. Persistent pyuria need to r/o TB. This may need potentially a kidney biopsy to r/o chronic pyelonephritis or interstitial nephritis.
- **Kidney Stones:** Single stones—need to rule out if metabolic cause—could donate, need to be counseled that risk of recurrence is 50% in five to seven years. Patient with bilateral stones or nephrocalcinosis, metabolic stones, are contraindicated.
- **Hyperuricemia:** Associated with decline in kidney function postdonation and should be discussed if patient has Hx of gout.
- **Malignancy:** Can donate if early stage, cured, and risk of transmission is rare.
- **CV risks major:** Major and intermediate risk factors are a contraindication, while minor risk factors can be individualized.
- **Acceptable donor renal function:** GFR ≥ 80 ml/min. But needs to be individualized to patient age and BMI. Lower GFR (sixty to eighty) in small people / people who are vegetarian or have low-protein diets (< 1 g /kg/ day) without other RF maybe acceptable but need close follow-up posttransplant. Low-protein diets can result in a low creat clearance—if not sure can sometimes trial a high-protein diet and retest. Projected decrease in GFR < forty in an eighty-year-old should be a contraindication.
- **Infectious disease:** Some are clear like HIV / Hep C; others can be treated and then offered. HOPE / EXPANDER trials have used DBD donors with HIV and Hep C donors.

- **Inheritable conditions that can affect donors:**
  - ***Alport syndrome*** (screen for sensorineural deafness and eyes / lens abnormalities and unexplained hematuria). X-linked recessive and 15% autosomal recessive.
  - ***Fabry disease***—X-linked recessive but heterozygote females will be affected too and at risk of ESRD.
  - ***Thin basement membrane disease***—although benign after a uninephrectomy, can strain kidney disease and progress to ESRD. Hard to sometimes differentiate histologically from Alport or IgA nephropathy. Presents as hematuria.
  - ***Strong FSGS** family* history may indicate an inherited form of glomerulonephritis.
  - ***SLE***—12% positive in primary family members. + ANA is associated with forty times risk of future SLE and is a C/I.
  - ***Sickle cell trait***—is a C/I in some centers—donor increased risk of medullary carcinoma / papillary necrosis and needs close surveillance.
  - ***APOL 1 gene mutation (G1 and G2)*** homozygous or compound heterozygous—in AA young donors, is associated with increased risk with future progression to ESRD and increased kidney allograft rejection by recipient. It is associated with increased risk of FSGS.

Assessments:

- **GFR:**
  - GFR most accurate and reliable measured by **isotope clearance (iothalamate clearance)** accepted 80 ml/min/m2 (adjusted by age)—not widely available.
  - **CrCl**—twenty-four-hour urine collection (tend to **overestimate**).
  - **eGFR**—using MDRD or Cockcroft-Gault (tend to **underestimate** but better than CrCl).

- Interestingly the **average of the MDRD + CrCl** was better than any of the individual tests (CG / MDRD / CrCl).
- **Proteinuria:**
  - Twenty-four-hour urine collection, > 250 mg/day—is a C/I.
  - Microalbuminuria assessment used to assess early sign of renal injury or if borderline proteinuria.
  - Orthostatic proteinuria—common in younger patients—is not a contraindication.
- **Anatomical:**
  - Contrast CT better than MRI.
  - Surgical preop and to r/o stone / malignancy.
  - Multiple vessels / collecting systems are not RF for graft survival / function.
  - Kidney size.
  - Right versus left—no difference in outcome; right will have shorter vessels.
  - **Renal cysts:** Which are acceptable versus high risk of malignancy:
    - **Bosniak classification**—based on CT imaging characteristics:
      - **One-half:** low risk (0% malignancy risk), simple to minimally complex cysts, nonattenuating, < 3 cm, thin few septa, well defined. Thin calcification if any.
      - **2F:** 5% risk of malignancy—may need serial US to evaluate.
      - **Three to four:** 55–100% malignancy risk not used—donor will need treatment.
    - US suspicion of **APKD** (adult polycystic kidney disease).
      - Patients with unknown family history, three or more unilateral or bilateral kidney cysts in those aged fifteen to thirty-nine.

        - Two cysts in each kidney in those at risk aged 40-59.
        - Less than or equal to four cysts in each kidney in at-risk patients ≥ sixty.
        - Patient who are young and at risk but with less cysts are not cleared yet; MRI may be more sensitive to pick up smaller cysts, and also genetic testing should be done. If both are negative, then they are cleared.

- **Immunologic assessment:**
    - A donors A1 / A2 subtyping needed.
    - HLA.
    - Paired exchange evaluation versus ABO incompatible desensitization plans.
- **Psychosocial evaluation:**
    - Coercion.
    - Alcohol / substance abuse / smoking.
    - Live Donors: Can be reimbursed for time off work / travel and child care.
    - Educational and billing coordinator.
- **Consent:**
    - All risks—UTI, retention, hernia, seroma, SSI, bleed, VTE, open conversion, death (0.02–0.04%).
    - Opt out at any time.
- **Operative Technique:**
    - Laparoscopic (including hand assisted) versus open.
        - 16% versus 13% higher than open complications.
        - Shorter stay and less analgesia with laparoscopic.

Kidney Back Table Principles

Back table principles:

- **Rule 1:** arterial and vein length should be the same.
- **Rule 2:** arterial branches may cross the vein anteriorly. (Check direction of artery path using probe.)
- **Rule 3:** always flush artery and vein to determine potential leaks.
- **Rule 4:** limit dissection around the ureter (blood supply to ureter).

Back table:

- Inspect the kidney for damage.
- Mark ureter, suture ends of vein and artery.
- Left kidney:
  - Tie off lumbar / adrenal and gonadal branches
  - Low on vein, smaller vein closer to the hilum.
- Artery:
  - Look for accessory artery.
- Don't dissect too close to hilum.
- Dissect fat but keep that close to ureters.
- Keep kidney submerged in cold preservative during back table.

Reconstruction artery:

- 18–30% vascular aberrations in general population and may need reconstruction.
- 1–2 mm accessory arteries to upper pole may supply 10–15% of kidney—may be difficult to preserve.

- Lower pole arteries must be preserved as they supply the ureter.
- Common Carrel patch for arteries 10 mm apart on common aortic patch.
- > 10 mm apart—sew two carrel patches together.
- Or two V-plasties with side-to-side anastomosis such that one common arterial orifice is formed.
- Or end to side if one vessel has uneven length +/− interposition autogenous graft gonadal vein of donor or epigastric artery of the recipient.
- Advantage of implanting arteries separately is preserved flow to kidney if one vessel is thrombosed, but disadvantage is prolonged ischemia time.
- Check for intimal dissection.

Multiple renal veins:

- Left most common.
- If vein is < one-third of main renal vein, it may be sacrificed.
- Short right renal vein—risks kinking thrombosis, difficulty sewing, unable to adequately check for bleeding postreperfusion. Use caval patch to reconstruct longer vein length.

Ureters:

- Damaged ureters are not repaired, usually just need to deal with a short ureter by sewing a ureteroureterostomy or bladder hitch.

Biopsy site:

- Biopsy site repair with five Prolene deep bites, not to tie too tight as it will tear with reperfusion. May use absorbable sutures if you believe collecting system is involved.

Kidney Transplantation and Surgical Procedures

Approach:

- **Retroperitoneal.**
- **Intraperitoneal** (children < 20–25 kg or multiple previous kidney Txp previously).

Kidney ipsilateral versus contralateral (depends on scars, calcification of iliac vessels).

Intraoperative pointers:
Repair peritoneal tears at time of identification, as they will only increase in size.

May achieve recipient iliac vein mobilization by ligating pelvic tributaries.

When vessel discrepancy:

- Longer vessel should be anastomosed distally

Contralateral organs:

- Left kidney—lies medially in right side; least kinking and is more anatomical.

Arteries > two cm apart will need reconstruction or plugged in separately or reconstructed.

Test clamp renal vein above anastomosis.

Arterial vasodilators—verapamil five mg instilled proximal to the renal artery. Topical papaverine.

Use diuretics—mannitol / Lasix—after vascular reconstruction is performed.

Ureteral anastomosis:

- Most common Lich-Giegor.
- Trim and spatulate ureter posteriorly.
- Stent use: Reduced complication but higher infectious risk and needs removal in four to six weeks.
- Drain use is variable.

Pathway Course:

This starts by first having an expectation for the transplanted kidney. If the donor kidney is a young kidney, with very short cold ischemia, one would expect for it to work immediately. So if postop the kidney does not match your expectation, then it's important to investigate why before even fascial closure. Factors: Is the lie of the kidney kinking the vessels? Is it a tight facial closure causing abdominal compartment? Are there vascular dissection or technical factors affecting the anastomoses?

Postop:

- **CNS:**
  - Analgesia: Patients will generally need a PCA.
- **CVS:**
  - **Blood pressure goals:** MAP ≥ 65 mmHg. It is better to keep the blood pressure slightly in the hypertensive side (SBP ≤ 160 mmHg) to allow better kidney perfusion.
    - Hypertension with BP above that goal: can be treated with Hydralazine IV PRN, Labetalol PRN IV, Metoprolol IV PRN. In extreme cases that are close to HTN urgency or emergency ≥ SBP 200 mmHg, the patient may need to be on a labetalol drip or a nicardipine drip.
    - If patient is known to be a patient with uncontrolled HTN, it is important to anticipate this postop and

quickly reinstate some of his meds. It is important not to use ACE or ARB early postop.

- **Hypotension:** R/o bleeding—Hb checks and JP drainage color and output.
  - Is patient adequately resuscitated? Look at total in / outs from OR record. Does patient need IVF bolus because they are dry?
  - Thymoglobulin: Can cause a cytokine-related vasodilatory effect and cause low BP. You can try to decrease the rate it's flowing by half or hold and see if this improves BP.
- **Respiratory:**
  - Patient will need to have a pulmonary toilet ordered.
- **GI:**
  - NPO—in case patient will need to go back to the OR for an emergency.
  - PPI to prevent gastric stress ulcers, especially if these patients are on steroids.
  - Stool softeners should start with diet.
- **Renal:**
  - **Does patient need dialysis?**
    - Are they volume overloaded, or do they have hyperkalemia? Is the allograft functional (i.e., will they respond to diuretics)?
    - Do they have AVF (is it still patent?) or a catheter for access that can be used? If you need to place an access, how safe is it (history of failed accesses)?
- **GU:**
  - Three-way or two-way foley:
    - Duration depends on bladder quality.
      - Good tissue duration of foley will be three days.
      - Poor tissue quality / friable—foley can stay seven to ten days.
    - Make sure, especially initial postop, that foley is not clotted off (due to fresh anastomosis bleed), especially if there is a sudden drop in urinary output.

Allograft that functions straight away: POD 0:

- Monitored bed, NPO, IVF—thirty cc/hr maintenance + (cc per cc replacement of UOP / hour with one-half NS or NS, depending on their sodium status). PCA, PPI, imaging postop—renal duplex to check on kidney) stat labs in recovery and check Q4 hours / Q6 hours, depending on how functional the allograft is. Replete electrolytes and HCO3 as needed; catch hyperkalemia before it's dangerously elevated. Heparin IV given intraop, so immediate HSQ is dependent on the risk of bleeding and clotting with patient risk factors. Maintain BP goals.

POD 1:

- Advance diet to clear liquid diet, stool softeners. Out of bed and pulmonary toilet. Resume home meds (if no contraindication), adjust BP meds. Stop PCA, remove arterial line, nonmonitored bed, change patients who are *pathway* to maintenance fluid. Start CNI +/− rest of induction doses over the coming days (depends on type of induction).

POD 2:

- Remove dressing, advance to regular diet, all PO meds, Hep-lock, Foley removal. Adjust BP and SSI management finalization.

POD 3:

- Remove JP < 50 cc/day. Adjust maintenance IS. Finalize BP and DM care.

Postoperative Surgical Complications

Early:

- **Bleeding / hematoma:**
  - Can present as shock / expanding hematoma on US (initial spread superiorly in retroperitoneum) → immediate re-exploration.
- **Vascular thrombosis:**
  - **Renal vein thrombosis:** Presents with **oliguria, hematuria,** and **pain.** Doppler—absent venous flow and reversal of arterial flow. Immediate reexploration.
    - Tx: anticoagulation.
    - Surgery: vessel control–like artery. Evacuate any hematoma, compartment compression release. If it's a living right renal vein, it's very friable and maybe explantation and preservative flow flushing is better than just doing venotomy and Uthrombectomy. Renal biopsy.
  - **Arterial thrombosis:** 2%, RF kinking, dissection, intimal flap, hypercoagulation, hypotension, high renal parenchymal resistance, obstructed inflow.
  - Tx: Immediate reexploration. Anticoagulate. Proximal and distal control of iliacs artery / vein. Clamp vessels, divide artery above anastomosis, complete thrombosis → explant, incomplete thrombosis → Fogarty embolectomy. Do renal biopsy.
  - Engorged, swollen kidney → capsulotomy and delayed facial closure.
- **Compartment syndrome:**
  - Hematoma, tight closure, PCKD. Remove cause +/– intraperitoneal window to leave kidney in.
- **Urine leak:** 1–3%.

- Ischemia versus technical.
- Early foley removal → outflow obstruction.
- Operative mgx if early and stented:
  - Foley, JP drainage if needed conservative.
  - Not improved → operative.

Late:

- **Lymphocele:** most are medial along lower pole of kidney.
  - < three cm doesn't need intervention
  - > three cm / compressive → aspirate +/– drain or sclerotherapy with either high-percentage alcohol or betadine.
  - Persistent (four to six weeks) despite drainage or two times aspirations need surgery (laparoscopic fenestration procedure use intraop US and slit should be five cm.
  - DGF and fluid overload should be corrected prior to surgical intervention.
- **Renal artery stenosis:**
  - Clinical: HTN, Bruit, CHF, Hypervolemia, impaired renal function.
  - Etiology: 40% fibrosis, 30% atherosclerosis, 20% kinking.
  - US:
    - Peak systolic velocity > 2.5 cm/sec along the renal artery.
    - Velocity gradient from stenotic to prestenotic area is more than two to one.
    - Marked distal turbulence with spectral broadening.
    - Prolonged acceleration time > 0.07 sec, diminished acceleration peak < 3 m/sec.
    - Parvus tardus wave forms proximal to stenosis.
    - Reduced RI < 0.5 renal parenchyma.
    - MRA can confirm stenosis

        - Angiographic confirmation: more than ten mmHg across the gradient of stenosis.
        - Tx: angioplasty (80% success)—stents limited data.
            - Surgical: higher ATN and graft loss postprocedure.
            - Anastomosis revision.
- **Ureteral stricture: 3%.**
    - Etiology:
        - Technical, ischemia, polyoma virus (BKV).
        - Direct nephroureterography or Lasix renogram if hydronephrosis is not significant.
        - Tx Balloon dilatation, stent placement.
            - Surgical if two interventions failed.
                - Distal injury: Ureterocystostomy.
                    - Psoas Hitch.
                    - Boari Flap.
                    - Ureteropyelostomy.
                - Ileal conduit.

Desensitization Protocols for ABO Incompatible and HLA Sensitized Patients

Alloantibody sensitization measured:

- **T-cell AHG (antihuman globulin) PRA:** historically not useful in telling B-cell sensitization and DSA.
- **T-cell AHG crossmatch:** positive considered a contraindication to transplant.
- HLA beads.
- **Flow cytometry crossmatch (FCXM):** allows detection of low-level noncytotoxic ab even if there is no cytotoxicity.
    - Negative FCXM: B-cell mean channel shift (MCS) < 130, T cell < 70 MCS.
- DSA levels using:
    - Luminex beads (array of HLA or a single antigen bead [SAB]): Measured as MFI (mean fluorescent intensity).
        - SAB Luminex beads with MFI > ten thousand is associated with ABMR.
        - Low risk DSA < five thousand MFI; moderate risk is five to ten thousand MFI, and High risk > ten thousand MFI.
        - DSA RIS score is used to assess risk. Zero points given for no DSA, two points if low-risk DSA < five thousand MFI, five points for every risk DSA five to ten thousand MFI, and ten points high-risk DSA > ten thousand MFI.
        - If DSA RIS > seventeen, it's considered contraindication.
    - **Acceptable for transplant after desensitization:**
        - Negative CDC in one to two or higher dilution,
        - FCMX with a shift of < 225 MCSs.

- DSA scores ≤ seventeen.
- In one study using these criteria reduced the ABMR rate to ~16% in the first year posttransplant.

Sensitized patients risk factors:

- Previous blood transfusions.
- Prior transplants.
- Pregnancies.
- Ten to twenty percent of patients will have a PRA > 10% with no risk factor.

Prevention of alloimmunization:

- Avoiding transfusions and pregnancy as much as possible.
- Performing transfusions under cyclosporine administration may decrease alloimmunization reported in two studies. Cyclosporine started four days prior to transfusion and continued one month after.
- Not ideal for predialysis patients as this may push them into dialysis or hyperkalemia.
- Leukocyte filtering of blood products.

Desensitization Protocols:

Is used for ABO incompatible patients or HLA highly sensitized patients with potential live donors. These protocols will lower the DSA titers, allowing potential transplant safely. Sometimes these protocols will need to be repeated posttransplant as "rescue" treatments for postop rejection.

- **IVIG:**
  - Role is neutralization of alloantibodies and consequential complement activation, inflammatory cytokine response, and inhibition of antibody production.

- It can also modify APC and B-cell activity. It leads to apoptosis of plasma cells and inhibits growth factors for B cells.
- Effects also T-cell proliferation with significant reduction in costimulatory and adhesion molecules.

Published Regimens:

- **High-dose IVIG 2 g/kg +/– Rituximab:**
    - Thirteen out of fifteen patients studied by Glotz et al. (European study) responded after repeated doses (three monthly doses) (success was defined as 50% reduction in PRA).
        - Two out of thirteen had live donors, rest were cadaveric.
        - Two out of thirteen lost grafts, rest had no rejection episodes up to one year follow-up.
    - NIH IGO2 study: Four months of three monthly doses of IVIG versus placebo. Patient continued with monthly IVIG perfusions for four months posttransplant.
        - Thirty-five percent of patients on IVIG were transplanted, and four out of sixteen IVIG patients had graft loss.
    - Khawaji et al.: IVIG given one month prior to transplant and one week prior to transplant. Rituximab given one week after the first dose. IVIG then given one week after the transplant.
        - Six year follow-up of fifty-three patients: 15% had rejection, but six-year graft survival was 90% and had GFR of 63.9 +/– 23.
        - Ninety-six percent patient survival.
- **Plasmapheresis (PP):** Half of DSA per run + low dose IVIG after each phoresis session (100 mg/kg) given to prevent hypogammaglobulinemia.
    - Montgomery et al.: 211/215 desensitized patients had kidney transplant, living donors.

        - Number of treatments varied to get a negative X-match and lower DSA. On average, patients received 4 ± 4 plasmapheresis sessions before transplant and 5 ± 4 plasmapheresis sessions after transplant.
        - MMF and tacrolimus were started with initiation of pheresis and continued posttransplant.
        - Increased patient survival was noted with desensitization versus patients who remained on dialysis and those who were wait-listed for a DDKT.
    - Khawaji et al.: One month prior to transplant IVIG (high dose), followed by rituximab dose a week later. Two weeks prior to transplant, plasmapheresis every other day times five sessions followed by IVIG dose. Transplant a week later followed by IVIG one week postop.
        - Six-year follow-up: Twelve out of fifteen = 80% had rejections. Graft survival was 76%, and patient survival was 84.6%
    - Schweitzer et al.: (Three pheresis sessions per week). Six sessions of plasmapheresis with IVIG low dose after each session, also included start on tacrolimus, MMF and prednisone. Posttransplant patients had daily OKT3 for ten days. OKT3 no longer in use.
- **Plasmapheresis versus IVIG:**
    - For titers 1:8–16 IVIG could not convert a positive T cell to negative crossmatch versus PP was able to.
    - Titers > 1:16 could not be negatively converted either way.
    - Titers 1:8 or below responded to desensitization.
    - Titers 1:2 were acceptable for transplantation.

Future role:

- **Tocilizumab:** IL-6 receptor monoclonal ab. Cedars-Sinai used it for IVIG + Rituximab-resistant patients. Given 8 mg/kg monthly up to six months. Five out of ten patients had a transplant. Continued posttransplant use has shown persistently low DSA MFI. More data is needed.

- **Eculizumab:** monoclonal ab inhibiting C5a. Although a Mayo Clinic study comparing the usual plasmapheresis method versus using Eculizumab (day zero, one, weekly for month, and then biweekly for one year posttransplant) showed similar graft and patient survival outcomes, it was not reproduced.
- **C1 esterase inhibitor:** no solid data yet to support its use.
- **Bortezomib**: when used in addition to IVIG and rituximab was only associated with modest DSA reduction.

Orandi et al.: evaluated outcomes of desensitization at twenty-two US centers. Assessments of patient and graft survival showed that attempts to desensitize patients with positive complement-dependent cytotoxicity crosshatches (CDC-CMX) showed poor long-term graft and patient survival compared with nonsensitized controls.

Paired donation alternative approach to desensitization.

Tolerance ablation: T-cell ablation and bone marrow suppression at time of kidney donation. T-cell tolerance, however, doesn't always result in B-cell tolerance.

A2 to B Kidney Transplants

A2 donors express low levels of A antigen on the cell surface and are less immunogenic toward anti-A Ig present in B blood group or O blood group recipients.

Adopted by new KAS in an attempt to improve equitable allocation to minorities from subcontinents who have a higher blood group B / O representation.

Select B recipients have equivalent (A2 to B) outcomes versus ABO compatible recipients.

Criteria includes two consecutive anti-A IgG titers < 1:8 and anti-A IgM/G titers ≤ 1:64. Titers above so are not eligible.

Titers should be checked postop transplant and in uneventful cases followed at discharge per institutional protocol.

Induction agents used in such transplant include thymoglobulin or altemtuzumab with a steroid taper. Although it is the opinion of the author that thymoglobulin would be more efficient at decreasing risk of antibody-mediated rejection.

Maintenance regimen per institution would include MMF, tacrolimus +/– prednisone.

Postop titers that elevated anti-A IgG titers > 1:8 and anti-A IgM/G titers ≤ 1:64 patients will need plasmapheresis daily for five days by postop day one + single dose IVIG (2 g/kg) + Rituximab (375 mg/m^2).

Outcomes:

- Published data has shown similar graft and patient survival at one year.

- Although divergence in two year graft function in A2 to B versus B to B 2.4 Cr mg/dL versus 1.4 Cr mg/dL (albeit not statistically significant Vanderbilt data), there is no data to look at three-year and five-year graft survival.
- In one study, 65% required plasmapheresis for elevated titers.
- Significant costs associated with A2 to B transplants.

Two-for-One Kidney Transplants and Use of Pediatric En Blocs

Estimated eight hundred unrealized pediatric donors annually (≤3 years or younger) only two to three hundred performed of these annually.

Two-for-one adult kidney transplants account for only 0.5% of deceased donor transplants, roughly sixty annually.

Also KDPI does not take into account dual kidneys and can be a negative labeling of the kidneys, with falsely high KDPI. KDRI is a better assessment.

For kidney donors < eighteen years of age, it's up to the recipient surgeon to decide whether the kidney can be split or used as en bloc.

For ≥ eighteen years of age criteria or dual kidney allocation, include at least two of the lower criteria:

- Donor ≥ sixty years old.
- CrCL < sixty-five ml/min on admission.
- Rising serum creat on retrieval > 2.5.
- Donor medical history of HTN/ DM.
- Renal biopsy showing moderate to severe glomerulosclerosis > 15% < 50%.

En bloc kidneys:

Patient weight and kidney size are better cutoffs to kidney use versus donor age.

Many centers use < 8 kg or kidney size < 6 cm as exclusions for en blocs.

Also recipient's contraindications criteria include:

- High weight > 200 lb. / BMI > thirty.
- High PRA (> twenty).

- Severe HTN.
- High risk of recurrent disease (e.g., severe FSGS), (these organs often show signs of hyperfiltration and so initial signs of glomerulosclerosis with associated proteinuria postop).
- Hypercoagulable (e.g., lupus) disorder.
- Sickle cell disease (increased risk sickling in small vessels).
- Abnormal bladder anatomically or functionally.

Surgical factors:

- UW solution is associated with less graft thrombosis versus HTK.
- Hypothermic pulsatile perfusion was associated with greater graft survival.
- Minimal dissection should be performed on backbench.
- Mainly closure of suprarenal aorta (it is desirable to have SMA cuff—any lower cuff closure can increase thrombosis risk extending to renal arteries) and superior renal cava.
- Infrarenal aorta and caval ligation of lumbar and mesenteric branches.
- Minimal renal hilum dissection as not to damage potential accessory vessels.
- Perinephric fat preserved so that this tissue can be used to fix kidney to surrounding structures and prevent torsion.
- Ureters sewn conjoint versus separate on stents.
- Prior to closure, important to get intraoperative US to make sure no torsion or compression factors during closure.
- Often daily US is performed, especially in presence of DGF to r/o perfusion-related issues.

Two-for-one adult kidney

If using the Cockcroft-Gault formula for the admission and terminal serum creatinine of the donor was:

- > 65 ml/min: single kidney was used.
- ≥ 30 ≤ 65 ml/min: dual was used.
- < 30 ml/min: declined.

Other important factors that are strong donor features for contraindication:

- DIC.
- Rhabdomyolysis.
- Large kidneys > 13 cm (space consideration).
- Complex anatomy (multiple vessels / ureters).
- Projected long CIT; this is often center dependent, but < forty hours is acceptable.
- Glomerulosclerosis > 35%; it is the author's recommendation that a MAPI scoring system be used to assess this. Scores > seven should not be used.

Recipient criteria:

- Should be closely matched for age of deceased donor (i.e., older).
- Low PRA.
- Space factor (small stature or presence of Polycystic kidneys were C/I).
- Vascular factors (no long segment of concentric atherosclerosis).
- Adequate bladder capacity to allow for two anastomosis.
- Not on anticoagulation.
- No history of thrombophilia

- Good cardiac history EF > 40–50%; no a-fib or severe valvular disease.
- No previous pelvic surgery or irradiation.

Often these organs are accepted with "full waivers" (i.e., if organs are not used due to any reason the acquisition costs will not be paid by the accepting center if they were not used).

"Waivers" can be "full" for any reason, "anatomical" (only gross damage incurred during procurement or abnormal anatomy not described previously) or "biopsy" (institutional read of biopsy or repeat biopsy worse than described on DonorNet or if not done on procurement).

Since these kidneys (two for one) are considered marginal they're often placed on pump as a tool to limit ischemia damage and to evaluate it. Pump numbers: flow rate > 60 ml/min and RI < 0.5 after a minimum of six hours on machine are considered minimal threshold. Exclusive discard based on pump numbers should be avoided and the picture considered, especially if there is discrepancy between kidney pumps.

Surgical options:

- Bilateral extraperitoneal, Gibson incision (increased time by one to two hours).
- Unilateral extraperitoneal.
- Lower midline intraperitoneal.
- Lower midline extraperitoneal.
    - With bilateral placement of kidney, left kidney should be placed left so that the longer vein can reach the deeper external iliac vein.
    - In a unilateral extraperitoneal approach, right kidney renal vein anastomosed to IVC and renal artery to common iliac artery.
    - Reperfusion of the right kidney is done before clamping the lower vessels for the left kidney transplant per usual approach.

- The superior kidney is placed laterally and the lower kidney placed medically.
- This saves an hour on dissection and also saves the opposite side for future need.
- Modifications can be done if venal reconstruction with IVC cuff on right renal vein can allow external iliac vein reach versus the IVC.
- Ureters can be sewn into bladder separate or conjoint with stents.

Perioperative care:

- Induction agents include thymoglobulin or alemtuzumab. "Marginal" donors at increased susceptibility to ischemia reperfusion injury and therefore antigenicity leading to early rejection risk; therefore, antibody depleting agent is preferable.
- Steroid taper.
- MMF, tacrolimus, and prednisone maintenance / per institutional protocol.
- Important for en-blocs to start tacrolimus low dose and go up slowly as it can cause vasoconstriction, especially in the small vasculature.
- Immediate heparinization or use of "vodu" (untitratable low dose) heparin has been described for en-bloc kidneys.
- ASA prophylaxis is started once postop risk bleed is minimal and prior to discharge.
- Close BP control is essential, especially in en-bloc to prevent anastomotic breakdown.

Outcomes:

- Peds en-bloc graft survival is an equivalent to living donor graft survival and is higher than SCDs.
- In some institutions (two for one), five year renal function was comparable to single SCD and superior to single ECD, which translated to a higher KDPI than advertised

on DonorNet (in one study mean KDPI was 83% but actual KDPI was 60%).

- Same DGF rates to SCD and ECD.
- When using a single kidney, you are roughly transplanting 50–60% of donor estimated creat clearance versus with dual adult kidney transplants, you are transplanting 70–80% of the donor renal functional capacity.

Use of Hepatitis C Viremic Kidneys in Non–Hepatitis C Infected Recipients

The risk of transmission from HCV NAT –ve donors with Ab +ve serology has not been reported to our knowledge. This shows that the donor was infected or exposed to Hep C but cleared and developed immunity later on. This type of donor is considered low risk for HCV transmission and should be offered to recipients after adequate education

Total of >1,500 procured organs with Hep C; 57% of these kidneys were utilized in 2016.

Thinker trial and Expander-1 showed success in transplanting kidneys from HCV + viremic donor into noninfected HCV recipients.

The donors were NAT+ and recipients NAT-ve.

Postop treatment of Hep C with antivirals resulted in complete Hep C eradication and with successful graft and patient survivals for one year equivalent to normal cohort.

In those initial trials, antiviral therapy was either started upon viremic changes in recipients (Thinker trial three to five days postop) or even at the time of transplant (Expander-1, first dose given immediately before transplant) with often DAA combinations depending on HCV genotype and for durations of twelve to sixteen weeks.

Current DAA are able to treat pan-genotypes of Hep C with shorter courses (eight weeks e.g., Mavyret).

There have been publications on using this outside research practice and clinically with great success with third parties (insurance companies) covering DAA costs, with 100% one-year patient survival, one-year graft survival and HCV cure rates by Molnar et al.

Key factors when considering this:

Patient thorough education and consent process with their ability to opt out.

Making sure recipients do not have a liver disease or are at risk of severe hepatic dysfunction (especially that in some nonresearch studies often treatment was started after a median of seventy-six days posttransplant weeks after transplant during which some had three fold AST elevations; one out of fifty patients developed fibrosing cholestatic hepatitis).

- Liver function evaluations in recipients:
  - Fibrosis 4 (FIB-4) score: age, AST, ALT, and plt calculations.
    - Score < 1.45 had 90% negative predictive value for advanced fibrosis.
    - > 3.25 had a 97% specificity and 60% predictive value for advanced fibrosis
    - Scores 1.45–3.25 should be further assessed with FibroSure test
  - FibroSure test: A blood test with several liver and markers, which predicts degree of fibrosis.
    - Graded zero to four: F1-portal fibrosis, F2-bridging fibrosis with few septa, F3-bridging fibrosis with many septa, F4-cirrhosis.
    - FibroScan: Using US to detect fatty liver and cirrhosis.
    - Liver biopsy: Ishak scoring to estimate severity of fibrosis.

Have a readily available hepatologist with quick postop referral to initiate and lead treatment in liaison with the transplant team.

Thorough research into the patient medical payer system to see approval rate for DAA.

Ideally treatment should be started as early postop as possible to decrease risk of inflammatory changes and immune changes that can affect DGF / acute rejection episodes and even infections like CMV/ BKV etc.

There are studies investigating use of DAA (direct acting antiviral drugs) preop and for three days postop with a decreased transmission rate of HCV (quoted < 10%).

Use of Hepatitis B positve Donor Kidneys

Advances in Hep B immunity has allowed us to reappraise the use of Hepatitis B–labeled kidneys.

Serology of Hep B, after immediate infection:

Initial HBsAg—surface Antigen is positive after four weeks of exposure.

Anti-HBc antibodies to core Hep B proteins appear one to two weeks after HBsAg. Ig subtypes:

- IgM—first six months of infection—marker of acuity.
- IgG—thereafter the six months—marker of chronicity.

Anti-HBs—surface antibodies develop to mark immunity, usually IgG, and persists indefinitely

Understanding Serology:

HBsAg (+) + persistent—active infection uncleared—highly infectious.

HBsAg (+) + anti-HBc IgM: acute infection—highly infectious.

HBsAg (+) + anti-HBc IgG: Chronic infection—infectious.

HBsAg (–) + anti-HBs: Immune to Hep B, vaccinated (passive immunity). Could also have been exposed to infection with anti-HBc too low to be picked up.

HBsAg (–) + anti-HBs + anti-HBc: Immune due to previous exposure or infection—active immunity.

Only anti-HBc (+): Carrier to Hep B with HBsAg titers too low to be picked up (< 5% of cases), has low-risk transmission in thoracic and kidney recipients but considered high in liver recipients.

HBV DNA: will show even before HBsAg is positive and to evaluate active replication in chronic patients / carriers.

Transplanting Hep B Labeled Kidney Risks and Management:

HBsAg (+) +/– anti-HBc IgM (+) Donor in nonimmune recipient / immune:

- Highly infectious, often reserved for extenuating stances of medical necessity.
- Immune and nonimmune patients have shown evidence of active infection after transplantation.
- Many institutions will not include nonimmune recipients or recipients with anti-HBs titers < 100 IU/ml.
- Recipients recommendation: HBIG IV infusion (10,000 IU) daily for first seven days postop and monthly for the first year.
- Lamivudine / entecavir antiviral PO daily for first year.
- Frequent surveillance of liver function and serology.

Anti-HBc (+) only donors:

- Important to further evaluate the donor status by looking at Ig subtype of anti-HBc. IgM—should be treated and managed analogous to HBsAg (+) organs (see above) regardless of anti-HBs status. Donor immunity with anti-HBs dies not eliminate risk of HBV transmission, but it merely confirms that the anti-HBc was not a false positive—this would also be confirmed in donors who had a liver biopsy during procurement. Donor HBV DNA levels should be sent.
- IgG—has low risk of transmission in thoracic and kidney transplants; 1–4% risk of seroconversion. Risk is significantly higher for liver organs.
  - Recipients who are nonimmune, Donor HBV DNA (+) / unknown:
    - HBIG—daily for seven days postop (first dose intraop) and continues for three to six months.

      Or alternatively…
    - Lamivudine / entecavir started at time of transplant and continued for twelve months.
  - Recipients are immunized or Donor HBV DNA (–):

- No additional treatment with frequent surveillance (q3 months).

Donor anti-HBs only:

- Donor was immune or vaccinated. Negligible risk of transmission.
- Routine liver function evaluation.

Reported outcomes:

- Similar patient and graft survival in donors with HBsAg (+) used for recipients HBsAg (–) with anti-HBs titers > 100 IU/ml in one retrospective study with fifty-eight-months mean follow-up.
- Same rejection rate versus noninfected donors.
- No biopsy changes with Hep B glomerulopathy
- Nonseroconverted.
- One study suggested in patients with titers anti-HBs > 100 IU/ml, HBV prophylaxis was not even necessary.

Important to not forget that, patients undergoing plasmapheresis for AMR; may need HBIG prophylaxis.

Increasing reports of lamivudine resistance.

Kidney Transplant: Induction Therapy and Protocols

Induction agent:

- Antilymphocyte antibody immunotherapy, parenterally given, short course.

Historical use:

- Metchnikoff in 1898 first described → Woodruff in 1963 first used clinically in skin grafts of animals.
- Starzl first used it in a kidney in 1967.
- Cosimi 1990 first to use OKT3 monoclonal antibody.

Only Basiliximab (Simulect) and Daclizumab (Zenapax) were FDA approved for induction use.

Types of induction agents used:

- ATGAM = Horse origin.
- ATG = Thymoglobulin (thymo) = rabbit origin, given as 3–6 mg/kg dose.
- Muromonab (CD3) = OKT3, off market.
- Daclizumab (Zenapax) = also discontinued.
- Basiliximab (Simulect), 20 mg given at induction and postop day four.
- Alemtuzumab (Campath), 30 mg given once at induction.

Rationale is to:

- Delay onset / reduce severity / minimize recurrence of acute rejection.
- Hope to allow tolerogenic response to donor alloantigen.
- Not expected to increase patient or graft survival rates.

Used in:

- High-risk recipients:
  - AA / re-transplant / SPK / sensitized.
- Delay use of CNI:
  - Expected DGF (ECD, DCD).
- Maintenance immunosuppression minimization:
  - Steroid / CNI withdrawal / avoidance.

Organ Specific:

- Highest for SPK → pancreas alone → kidney.
- Least used for liver → lung

Use trends:

- Thymo / Campath increasing
- Simulect / Zenapax decreasing

Use did not affect the five-year graft survival in both DD (66 → 70%) versus LD (80 → 80%) comparing trials in 2001 versus 2004.

Low Risk:

- 1997 Study: showed Simulect induction agent has lower biopsy-proven rejection at six months and one year (30% versus 44%), but same patient survival / graft survival / PTLD/ infection rates versus placebo.
- 1998 **Daclizumab** → similar to Simulect.

High Risk:

- **2006 ATG versus Simulect**—Same death / graft loss and DGF rates but lower biopsy proven rejection 15.6% versus 25%.
- Higher leukopenia and infection risk with ATG versus Simulect but same PTLD.
- **Campath, aka altemtuzumab**—humanized monoclonal anti CD52, which affects complement activation or cell-mediated cytotoxicity → peripheral lymphopenia → remains low for about a year.

- **Campath versus ATG** (6.0 mg /kg/d):
  - Thymo versus Campath similar biopsy proven rejection (13% versus 9.5%)
  - Infection rate same except respiratory infections higher in thymo patients (23%) versus (7%) Campath.

- **Rituximab: use as part of induction agent in high PRA or retransplants/ DSA:**
  - Van den Hoogen et al.: showed low risk patient had no higher benefit with the addition of a single dose of rituximab at induction. (280 patients, prospective double blind study), results reached statistical significance.
    - Patients with higher immunologic risk actually had a lower rejection rate—17.9% versus 38% with $p = 0.06$.
    - More patients had neutropenia (24.3% vs 2.2%) but similar infection rates even at the four-year follow up.
  - Another study comparing:
    - (9 mg/kg of thymo versus 7.5 mg/kg of thymo) + (1 dose of rituximab versus 7.5 mg/kg of thymo) + (four doses of Bortezomib versus 6 mg/kg thymo + (one reduced dose rituximab 200 mg/m2) + (four doses of Bortezomib).
    - Showed similar risk of rejection in all and did not have enough power to merit one way or the other (only ten patients in each arm).

Conclusion:

- Tailor to organ type / recipient risk factor / quality of donor organ.
- Low risk: Simulect or low dose thymo (3–4.5 g/kg/d).
- High risk: High dose thymo (6.0 mg/ kg/d) versus Campath.
  - May consider in high risk immunologic patients the use of B-cell depletion with rituximab.

	peat dose POD4, 500mg MP given POD 0 and 250mg MP POD4 + Low dose tacrolimus + MMF. Group C: Daclizumab 1mg/kg (POD0)4 doses- each dose every 2 weeks., 500MP x3 doses and then weaned + Tacrolimus +MMF.	1 month and 4-6ng/ml 2-6months) and MMF (500mg bid) dose (steroid free)					Group B= 88%, Group C= 85%	Group B= 74%, Group C= 82%	in all 3 groups		related to the lower trough levels of CNI and MMF.
2003 NIH	Group 1: 30mg Campath, MP taper from 500mg to 0 by POD 5 + Tacrolimus + MMF. Group 2: 30mg Campath, MP taper from 500mg to 0 by POD 5 + Belatacept + MMF. Group 3: Simulect 20mg on POD 0 and 4, Same MP taper Tacrolimus Transitioned to Belatacept).	Group 1: Tacrolimus + MMF, Group 2: Belatacept (10mg/kg - POD0,4,28, 56,84 and then 5mg/kg every 4 weeks and MMF. Group 3: Tacrolimus slowly weaned troughs 8-12 (1 st month, 5-8 (2nd month), 3-5 (3rd month) and then stopped. Belatacept (10mg/kg - POD0,4,28, 56,84 and then 5mg/kg every 4 weeks and MMF	none	all types 6:6:7	19	3 yr	Group 1=70%, Group 2= 50%, Group 3= 100%	100% in all groups	Group 1/2= 1 BKV, Group 3= 3 BKV, no PTLD in any group	Group 1= 50% group 1 rejection episode. >300 days out. Group 2 had 33% rejection but had 4 recurrent episodes. Group 3= 71% had rejections, but upto 6 episodes.	Group 2 study enrollment (Campath + Belatacept + MMF) stopped due to increased observerd vascular thrombosis episodes. Higher ACR in belatacept groups
2003 Kirk et al	MP500mg + Campath 30mg intraop	Belatacept 10mg POD1, 3,7,14, (Q14 days x 4), (Q monthly till month 6 and then 5mg monthyly thereafter vs Sirolimus POD 1 trough 8-12ng/ml for first year. Randomized to donor bone marrow infused on POD7	Sirolimus trough 3-8 ng/ml after 1 year. At one year offered to wean to belatacept monotherapy / off all IS or continue same	LD	20	3 yrs	100%	100%	BKV 10/20- 2 SV40 on biopsy but no nephropathy, low level EBV 5/20- self resolving CMV 1/20	3/20- BANF 1B or lower occuring >6 months on routine biopsy	All who choose off all IS- had a ACR or DSA (4-7 months after)- requiring treatment and dual maintenance therapy. Patients who didn't get bone marrow did as well as those who did get it.
2003 BEST study	All Groups had 500mgMP intraop pre induction, POD1- 500mgMP, POD2- 250mgMP, POD3- 125mg, POD4-80mgPred, POD5-60mg pred- None thereafter: Group1: Campath (30mg) intraop + (belatacept +MMF), Group 2: Thymoglobulin (4-6mg/kg) total by POD5-10, + (belatacept + MMF), Group 3: Thymoglobulin (4-6mg/kg) total by POD5-10 + (Tacrolimus + MMF)	Group 1: Belatacept (10mg at POD 1, 5,14,28,56,85 snd then 5mg/kg monthly thereafter+ 1 gMMF or MF, Group 2: Belatacept (same as above) + MMF, Group 3: Tacrolimus (8-12ng/ml target for 1st month and thereafter 5-10ng/ml target) and MMF (as above)	none	All types 107:104:105	316	1yr	Group 1= 1 death, Group 2= 3 deaths, Group 3= 1 death	1 CAN in Group 3. 1 PNF in group 2	Same infectious risk in all 64% vs 72% vs 66% NSS, 0 PTLD in all	G3 had lowest biopsy proven rejection and ACR(5% vs 17 G1, 23 G2) P 0.024, G2 was highest.	Conclusions: Group 2: (thymo + bela had higher BK viremia but without nephropathy with 0.09SS (20% vs 9.5% (G3) vs 11.2% (G1)). Kidney function in eGFR was satistically similar in all groups. Days to 1st BPAR were same in all groups. G3 had satistically significant lower BPAR and ACR and was milder (Banf 1b or below). G2 highest BPAR and ACR and highest Banf 2A and above) NODAT slightly elevated in Thymo + tacro group.

All these trials were done mainly on low risk PRA recipients

PS= Patient survival
GS= Graft Survival
LD= Living donors
DD= Deceased Donors

ACR= Acute cellular rejection
ABMR= Antibody mediated rejection
NR= Not recorded

PNF= Primary non function
Total N= total number of patients in trial
CAN= Chronic Allograft Nephropathy

published study year	Inuction Regimen	Maintenance regimen	long term changes	Donor type	Total N:	F/u duration	PS	GS	Infectious risks	ACR /ABMR	Notes
2003 Kirk et al	500mg -60mg (tapering) Methylpred + (0.3mg/kg Campath) Preop doses x 3 or (1 preop + 3 postop doses)	None	none	LD	7	1 yr	100%	100%	NR	100%- ACR	all developed ACR within 1 month. Campath alone is not sufficient for tolerance
2003 UW	500mg Methylprednisone + 20mg Campath (Intraop), Repeat dose POD 1	Rapamycin Monotherapy (trough 8-12ng/ml)	no change	All types.	24	1 yr	100%	96.40%	NR	12.5% -25% ABMR, 12.5% ACR (Banf 2a or below)	Most rejections occurred <1 month and all of them with rejection were switched after treatment to (MMF,FK, pred maintenance)
2003 UW	500mg Methylprednisone preop + 20mg IV Campath (intraoperative), POD 1 Repeat dose of MP and Campath + 1.5mg/kg thymoglobulin	Steroid taper over 14 day period + Rapamycin same as above goal.	no change	LDKT	5	1 yr	100%	100%	NR	40% all ACR(2a or below)	
2003 UPMC	1000mg Methylprednisone preop + 30mg IV Campath + 1000mg methylprednisone (prior to reperfusion)	Monotherapy Tacrolimus target 10 ng/ml	Tacrolimus reduced to daily dose at 100 days x 4 months and every other day if clinically well.	LD	205	1.4 yrs	98.60%	91.20%	0- CMV, 1.5% BKV, 0 % PTLD	10% in 1 yr (peaked after 6 months), 93.8% were BANF 2a or bellow	10% switched to combination (MMF + pred) or Sirolimus due to ACR
2003 Kaufman et al	500mg methyl pred , 30mg Campath or Simulect (dosing not specified), Methylpred 250mg POD 1, 125 POD 2	(steroid free) tacrolimus and MMF	no change	All types 123:155	278	30 months	96% camp vs 99% Simulect	99% for both	4% CMV , 1.5% PTLD	14.9% Campath vs 13.5% Simulect	Simulect had higher early rejection rate (72% within 1st 2 weeks), the late Campath rejections maybe related to lower MMF and prgraf dosing
2003 Kirk et al	0.3mg/kg Campath on days -1, +1,+3,+5 + Predosed with tapering, steroids starting at 500MP to 60mg. Deoxyspergualin armed into Days -1->12 or POD 12->25 (1st dose 4mg /kg rest 2.5mg/kg	none	none	LD	5	2 yrs	100%	100%	0	all developed ACR <1 month	Patients developed severe neutropenia and thrombcytopenia requiring lower dosing of deoxyspergualin, mild cytokine release like symptoms, 1 wound dehiscence. All patients needed ACR treatment- 4/5- steroids bolus treatment, 1 patient needed OKT3. They were then placed on monotherapy of sirolimus or tacrolimus.
2003 Flechner et al	500Methylpred Pre campath. Campath 30mg Intraop and POD 1	MMF 1 g BID + sirolimus 8-12ng/ml trough (steroid free)	none	14 LD: 8 DD	22	15.9 months	95.40%	86.30%	9% CMV, 0 PTLD	36% had Acute rejection (8/22), 2/8 (25%) ABMR, rest ACR, 1/8- had 2B Banff rest were lower, 6/8 75% developed ACR <3 months of transplant	2 patients developed severe URI leading to one patient death and the loss of 2 grafts.
2003 Ciancio et al	Group A =Thymo 1mg/kg/day= 7 days= total 7mg/kg, 500 MP x3 doses and then weaned + Tacrolimus + MMF. Group B= Campath 0.3mg/kg POD0 and re-	Group A/ C: Tacrolimus (8-10 ng/ml trough), MMF 1g bid, pred. Group B: lower tacrolimus (4-7 ng/ml @	none	DD 30:30:30	90	39 months	Group A= 85%,	Group A= 81%,	27% infectious hos-pitalizations	Group A= 20%, Group B= 23%, GroupC= 23%	Although steroid free at 39 months, Group B had higher CAN, maybe rel

Minimization of Calcineurin Inhibitors (CNI)

CNI = (Tacrolimus [FK] and cyclosporine [Cys])

Chronic allograft injury is due to:

- Chronic antibody rejection versus CNI injury.

Effects of CNI:

- **HTN:** (Cys worse than FK)
  - Increased sympathetic neural activation.
  - Decreased production of vasodilators (NO, prostaglandins, etc.).
  - Increased vasoconstrictors (endothelin, thromboxane, RAS).
  - Increased renal vascular vasoconstriction
  - Increased sodium and water retention.
- **DM:** New onset diabetes > 40%, impair beta cells of pancreas.
- **Dyslipidemia:** especially hypertriglyceridemia.
  - FK alone lowers dyslipidemia but with steroids causes increased dyslipidemia.
  - Sirolimus is the worst and also Cys.
- **Increased malignancy risk:**
  - However, sirolimus is associated with decreased incidence of cancer.

Pathophysiology:

- Increased vasoconstrictors / decreased vasodilators / Increased sympathetic activity / activation of renin angiotensin system / vascular smooth muscle necrosis → hyaline deposition → narrow the lumen.

- Local ischemia → free radicals → tubular injury → interstitial fibrosis → upregulation of TGF-B expression → fibrosis.
- Plt aggregation → thrombotic microangiopathy (TMA) a syndrome that includes a spectrum of TTP and HUS.

Key Features on Biopsy:

- Peripheral nodular **arterial hyalinosis**, with luminal narrowing.
- **Focal segmental glomerulosclerosis**.
- Isometric **tubular vacuolization**.

At one year 50% of biopsies showed CNI toxicity, and at ten years 100% from biopsy evidence.

Protocols and trials:

Avoidance: (Daclizumab induction followed by MMF and steroids only → higher rejection).

CNI withdrawal:

- **CAESAR trial:** Withdrawal over four months of CNI (Cys) → higher rejections without improvement in renal function. Needed low-dose CNI (Cys).

CNI reduction:

- **ELITE-Symphony trial:** Regimen (Cys + MMF + steroid) versus (Daclizumab induction + MMF + steroids + (either low-dose Cys or low-dose tacrolimus versus low-dose sirolimus).
  - The low-dose tacrolimus had a more superior graft function at twelve months and lower BPAR (12.3%) versus 25% (low-dose / standard-dose Cys) versus 30% in Sirolimus group.

CNI replacement: With:

- mTOR (sirolimus / everolimus) or (Belatacept [CTLA4 fusion protein]).
  - **Sirolimus:**

- **CONVERT Trial:** Patient on standard CNI regimen for 6–120 months posttransplant with GFR 20–40 ml/min or > 40 ml/min were randomized to CNI conversion to sirolimus versus continue CNI.
  - Patients with GFR > 40 had slightly **better GFR** but no difference in graft function or survival. Also **similar acute rejection**. And **lower malignancy**.
  - **Higher discontinuation** rates on sirolimus use with wound healing and diarrhea and worse outcomes for patients with GFR < 40 ml.
- **Everolimus:**
  - **ASCERTAIN Trial / TRANSFORM Trial:**
    - Everolimus versus 90% reduced CNI + low-dose Everolimus versus CNI continuation.
  - **No GFR difference, higher discontinuation** in everolimus group due to SE (diarrhea / anemia / aphthous ulcers). Lower viral infections in everolimus + reduced CNI group versus CNI group.
- Ferguson et al.:
  - Thymo standard induction in all study arms:
  - (Belatacept + MMF) versus (tacrolimus + MMF) versus (belatacept + sirolimus).
  - All had similar graft function
  - No statistical significance, but belatacept + sirolimus had numerically a rejection rate equivalent to tacrolimus group and a slightly higher GFR.

- **BENEFIT study:** (Simulect induction, CNI versus less-intense belatacept versus high-intensity belatacept).
  - Belatacept given as 10 mg/kg IV induction → day five, week two, four, eight, twelve. Later dose decreased to 5 mg/kg monthly.
  - Higher GFR at three years in CNI-free group.

- Higher acute rejection—but no difference in graft survival.
- Higher PTLD in belatacept.
- Subjects on belatacept have better allograft function at three years.

- **BENEFIT-EXT (extended):**
  - Same as trial above but on recipients of ECD.
    - Similar findings to the above.
    - **Improved CVD profile:** BP (lower by 5–10 mmHg) and lipid profile and NODAT (new onset diabetes after transplant) in belatacept group.
- **ELEVATE Study:**
  - Simulect induction. CNI switch to everolimus at ten to fourteen weeks:
    - eGFR same versus CNI at twelve and twenty-four months, but initially higher in everolimus group at nine months.
    - eGFR everolimus better than CsA at twenty-four months, sixty-four versus fifty-three.
    - Higher proteinuria and UPC ratio with everolimus at twenty-four weeks and in fact, 15% of which were everolimus-adverse S/E.
    - Everolimus noninferior endpoint in graft loss, > 1B BPAR, death versus CNI.
    - Higher rejection with everolimus (most mild 1, 2A) rare 2B versus CNI. FK and the same as CsA rejection rate also seen in the ZEUS trial.
    - AMR rare in both groups but higher AMR in everolimus by twelve months but not at twenty-four months.
    - More prominent DSA de novo for class 1 than class 2 for everolimus (teens) versus < 5% CNI.
    - IFTA on biopsy at twelve / twenty-four months, same for all groups.

- LVMI same for all groups, less cardiac events in everolimus groups at twelve months but same for all groups by twenty-four months.
- Adverse SE pyrexia, peripheral edema, mouth ulceration in everolimus. Less diarrhea with CsA but higher triglyceride and creat.
- NODM 10% for everolimus versus CNI (higher for FK versus CsA).
- CMV 4% everolimus versus 6.1% CNI.
- BKV 3.8% everolimus versus 9% CNI.
- Malignancy 2.8% everolimus versus 4.7% CNI.
- Discontinuation—most happened in everolimus groups second to allograft rejection.

- **CRADLE Trial:**
  - At 4-6 weeks pediatric de novo transplants were randomized into:
    - (everolimus + low dose tacrolimus+ steroid withdrawal at 6 months) vs (tacrolimus + MMF+ low dose prednisone)
    - At 36 months both groups had similar graft function and BPAR.
    - Everolimus group also had lower de novo DSA at 1 and 3 years.
    - Improved height growth in the everolimus groups esp. attributed to steroid withdrawal.
    - Everolimus group had a lower CMV infection rate at even 36 months (7.7% vs 18.6%).

Excel sheet with different studies.

In Conclusion:

The chronic CNI nephrotoxicity concerns have led to trials substituting CNI from the start of transplant or replacing after a period post-transplant or reducing its dosage when combined with another agent.

mTOR alternatives and belatacept are good options when concerned about CNI-related nephrotoxicity or high IS-related viral infections / cancer but should be tailored to patient needs and risks (i.e., wound healing, GI side effects, EBV status and belatacept risk of PTLD).

Tacrolimus rejection rates are lower when compared to belatacept or sirolimus based regimens, but without significant graft survival changes.

Depleting induction (thymo / Campath) has negated some of the early rejection fears seen with belatacept in earlier studies; nonetheless later rejection continues to be a concern.

Early steroid withdrawal is safe but should be addressed with caution in high-risk groups like high PRA, FSGS, or autoimmune cases.

Delayed Graft Function (DGF)

DGF: Defined by the need for dialysis within first week of transplant.
(very dichotomous / practice variation).

Alternative definition:

- **Creat reduction ratio (CRR2) % on day two.**
  - Immediate graft function if ratio > 30%, DGF defined as ≤ 30%.
    - Studies showed that dialysis-dependent or nondialysis-dependent DGF have poor five-year graft survival, and so HD is not a good (sensitive) marker.
- S Cr > 3 mg/dl on day five.
- Time S Cr to drop by 50%.

Etiology:

- Circulatory pressure
- Mechanical
- Immunologic
- Medications, TMA, CNI
- Recurrent disease (HUS / FSGS)
- ATN-DGF

Ischemia—reperfusion injury:
RF: DCD, ECD, high-terminal creat, long CIT, warm ischemia time, recipient heart failure, HLA-mismatch, donor and recipient obesity.
Incidence: (2–50%) practice based.
Difficult to test as DGF definition, not accurate and variable.

DGF associated with worse five year graft survival, 67% versus 89% (non-DGF), but MAPI score showed that DGF should not be used as a factor for five-year long-term survival. It is associated with increased costs, longer hospitalization, and increased morbidity. Ischemic reperfusion injury is believed to upregulate HLA and increase acute rejection risk.

MAPI (Maryland Aggregate Pathology Index) score: Looked at ECD kidneys with mean CIT thirty-three hours, (80% were > twenty-four hours).

- Score range zero to fifteen; a good score is zero to seven (had 95% five-year survival), eight to eleven (63% five year) is intermediate, and twelve to fifteen is worst (53%).
- Preimplantation biopsy correlated with long-term survival.
- DGF was present in 52% of those studied kidneys.
- ECD and DGF were not independent RF for poor five year outcome when looking at the pathologic score.

Prevention and management:

- Mannitol use / limit WIT / CIT / BP control.
- One RCT showed use of low-dose dopamine in donor did lower DGF rate (very small and weak study).
- Use of CCB to decrease DGF, was weak and low-quality study based.
- Prevention solutions HTK and UW were superior to (EC) Euro-Collins solution with lower DGF rates.
- Pump perfusion superior to cold storage with lower DGF / lower duration of DGF / PNF. But one-year graft function was the same.
- Allow use renal dosing of meds.
- Keep CVP > eight postoperatively.
- Induction agents use to delay CNI use (controversial of CNI causes DGF versus delays the recovery phase of DGF). It is crucial, however, to provide sufficient immunosuppression as patients are at increased risk rejection in the first one to twelve weeks posttransplant.
- Biopsy on day ten if graft function does not improve: C4d staining.

Postoperative Renal Dysfunction

Defined as:

- > 20% increase in creat rise.

Etiology:

- **Prerenal:**
    - Most common.
    - Hypovolemia / shock / third spacing.
    - ACEi → prerenal azotemia / CNI toxicity (new meds started that interact with CNI, e.g., CCB).
    - Acute thrombus / abdominal compartment syndrome.
    - Dx: FENA < 1%, FE Urea if patient has been using diuretics.
    - Tx: volume challenge / crystalloids / colloids / Tx shock, stop medicine.
- **Renal—Intrinsic:**
    - ATN, acute rejection, infection, GN (glomerulonephritis).
    - ATN:
        - Toxic (contrast / meds, e.g., CNI, IVIG, sucrose based / aminoglycosides).
        - Ischemic causes.
    - Dx:
        - Casts in urine, FENA > one, Bx, KIM 1—kidney injury markers—still under investigation.
        - **Acute rejection:** Bx, granzymes, perforins biomarkers.
        - Cultures.
        - **BKV:** Biopsy / urine / serum PCR.
        - **Allergic interstitial nephritis:** Bactrim / PCN / cephalosporins seen as eosinophils on biopsy.

        - Tx stop drug + short corticosteroids 1 mg/kg/day quick taper one to two weeks.
        - **HUS / FSGS:** Biopsy, elevated **UPC ratio**.
    - Tx: reverse cause + supportive care. *Lasix does not speed recovery of ATN.*
- **Postrenal:**
    - Ureteral:
        - Upper: stones / tumor / clot / fluid collection compressions.
        - Lower: stones / strictures—ischemia / dehiscence / PTLD / collection compressions / obstructed stents.
    - Bladder neck:
        - Clot / tumor / catheters blocked.
    - Urethral.
- Dx: US, CT.
    - Hydronephrosis significant: pyelogram / nuclear imaging
- Tx: relieve the obstruction.

Kidney Transplant Outcomes

Living Donor > SCD > ECD > DCD (SCD > ECD)

Marginal donor kidneys are better than remaining on dialysis.

Who benefits from ECD versus wait for SCD:

- > 40 years of age / OPO long waiting time 1,350 days / OPO with short waiting time who are diabetic.

MAPI Score and KDPI are better evaluations of donor quality than merely using ECD criteria (Please review kidney donor selection).

Chronic allograft nephropathy (CAN) = Chronic allograft dysfunction = IFTA: interstitial fibrosis / tubular atrophy, no specific cause:
Causes of Renal graft loss in first year:

- CAN 40%.
- Death 30%.

Serum creat: no accurate and sensitive for GFR dysfunction.
Proteinuria > 500 g/day had worse graft prognosis
RF:

- Antigen dependent: Acute rejections / de novo HLA versus non-HLA antibodies.
- Antigen independent: Donor age / dose of nephron / nephrotoxic drugs / HTN / CNI / HLD / CMV.

Maintenance of graft goals:

Control: HLD—statins / TG—gemfibrozil / HTN (< 130/80) / Proteinuria >300 mg / 24 hr.—ACEi / ARB / DM.

- CNI dose reduction.
- CNI → mTOR (not recommended in proteinuria).

Prevention of Coronary Artery Disease in kidney Transplant Recipients

CVD is 20–1,000 higher in chronic kidney disease versus the general population.

Highest especially in diabetics and due to a sedentary lifestyle that comes from fatigue.

CVD among transplant recipients had 40% cumulative incidence over ten years.

Risk factors for recipients:

- DM
- HTN
- Dyslipidemia (lipid profile similar to those with CKD on PD)
- Smoking (30% risk of CVD events versus 15% in nonsmokers)
- CKD: increased risk of calciphylaxis and vascular calcification. (Aim for calcium x phosphorus product to be < 55 mg^2/dL to help minimize this.)
- Hyperhomocysteinemia: folic acid replacement on risk reduction is inconsistent in studies.
- Chronic inflammation: main sources are poor dentition, obesity, and vascular access–related inflammation. Associated with worse graft outcomes and CVD. Obesity is associated with elevated CRP and IL-6.
- Anemia: EPO have been attributed to endothelial dysfunction and thrombosis and hence CAD.

Risk factors posttransplant:

Highest CVD risk in the first three months and highest in the first thirty days.

- **Volume status:** especially with increasing DGF.
- **Surgical stress and demand ischemia.**

- **Intraop fluid resuscitation:** overzealous or too little.
- Acute rejections / posttransplant lymphoproliferative disorders are associated with increased HR for CVD.
- **New-onset diabetes after transplant (NODAT):** 30% of recipients develop this by the first year. Increased risk with patients with metabolic syndrome.
- **Metabolic Syndrome is a cluster of the following:**
  - BMI > thirty, waist circumference for men forty inches, women thirty-five inches, serum TG > 150 mg/dL, HDL < 50 mg/dL / < 40 mg/dL in men, fasting glucose > 110 mg/dL, or BP > 130/85 mmHg.
  - It is similar to type 2 DM—combined insulin insufficiency and resistance. Related to use of glucocorticoids and CNI (worst with tacrolimus versus cyclosporine) due to direct β islet cell toxicity.
  - Steroid withdrawal strategies: Midtvedt et al. showed supraphysiologic steroid reduction from 16 mg/day to 9 mg/dl was associated with 25% improved insulin sensitivity versus 5 mg/day withdrawal had no effect. Select patients can undergo early steroid withdrawal without increased risk of rejection.
  - Weight loss and diet counseling are the first steps. Close involvement of a diabetologist, with insulin, as best for acute hyperglycemia.
  - Thiazolidinediones (e.g., pioglitazone) / rosiglitazone promote insulin sensitivity, enhance β cell function, and reduce CV complications—safe on kidney and minimal effect on CNI. Associated with edema and weight gain.
  - Meglitinides (e.g., repaglinide) was as effective as rosiglitazone with less hypoglycemia than sulfonylureas. Dose needs to be adjusted with CKD.
  - Exenatide (glucagon like peptide 1 receptor)—not studied on transplant recipients. Sitagliptin (DPP-4) — no long-term studies on recipients.
  - Metformin is contraindicated.

- Diabetes screening after transplant is recommended weekly for first four weeks, then at months three, six, and twelve and then annually according to KDIGO.
- **Chronic meds:** CNI leads to intimal hyperplasia, HLD, and HTN. mTORi—can lead to significant HLD. CNI and steroids contribute to NODAT.
- **HLD:** due to meds, diet liberation, and residual CKD (stage two to three).

Risk Factor Modification:

- HTN: posttransplant 85% still HTN, aim < 135/80 mmHg (per KDIGO guidelines).
  - β blockers recommended in those with known CVD. May also reverse CNI related headaches. Short acting labetalol is used in early periop period, often replaced by atenolol or metoprolol.
  - Dihydropyridine calcium channel blockers (e.g., nifedipine XL—rapid onset / amlodipine [takes seven days to reach steady state]) had an improved GFR by 12 mL/min versus ACEi (it counteracts CNI vasoconstrictive effects). Can lead to edema, headaches, and gingival hyperplasia. ACEi and CCB effect on left ventricular mass was no different in one study.
  - Nondihydropyridines (diltiazem and verapamil): associated with CNI interactions, often reserved to those with arrythmias.
  - ACEi / ARB CVD benefits are met with concerns of graft dysfunction, hyperkalemia, and effects worsened with renal artery stenosis. It's first line for patients with erythrocytosis, often useful in proteinuric patients. Not commonly used early postop due to risk of hyperkalemia and worsening graft dysfunction but no real contraindications for this.
  - Other agents—clonidine (fast acting, can lead to rebound HTN), hydralazine, minoxidil, and diuretics.

- HLD: ALERT-Ext trial showed CVD benefit with use of Fluvastatin.
  - Statins result in 15–30% lowering of cholesterol, LDL, and TGs.
  - Goal is for total cholesterol < 200 mg/dL, LDL < 100 mg/dL, TG < 150 mg/dL.
  - Amlodipine combined with simvastatin associated with toxicities.
  - Rhabdomyolysis and liver dysfunction side effects can occur with statins.
  - Triglyceride management: dietary control followed by niacin (first line), fibrates as second agents.
- Antiplatelet: Aspirin—cardioprotective.
- Smoking cessation:
  - Nicotine replacement and Chantix use, although not studied in transplant recipients, seem to be safe. Ideally cessation should start prior to transplant.
- Diet and exercise: weight gain due to dietary liberation and improved taste and less as a result of use of steroids. Exercised is associated with VO2 max, and in one study thirty exercise sessions lowered IL-6. Dietician and exercise psychologists are important.

Hematologic Surveillance Posttransplant

Anemia: complete workup: *CBC (with retic), blood smear, ferritin, transferrin saturation, folate, iron and B12 levels, haptoglobin, serum bilirubin, LDH, Coombs test, Parvovirus B19 PCR, bone marrow biopsy.*

- **Microcytic:** surgery related, bleeding, phlebotomy, and hemodilutional, iron deficiency (Ferritin < 200 ng/ml, transferrin saturation < 20%).
  - Transfuse to goal Hb > 8 g/dL, especially if symptomatic.
  - Iron replacement IV, replacement avoided in active infection.
  - Erythropoietin stimulating agents (EPO or darbepoetin (longer acting) C/I in uncontrolled HTN, active bleeding or stroke.)
- **Macrocytic:** B12 / folate deficiency. Do not replace folate in B12 depleted patients as this can lead to severe neurological changes.
- **Hemolytic:** Passenger lymphocyte syndrome: Hemolytic process due to use of incompatible blood products like an O donor to A recipient. often self-limiting. Coombs test to rule out autoimmune cause.
- **Red cell aplasia:** unresponsive to Epo. ELISA test not great at picking up Ig due to immunosuppression. Treated with IVIG successfully but has 25% recurrence.
- **Meds:**
  - MMF, azathioprine—profound bone marrow suppression.
  - ATG, Campath—sudden Hb drop.
  - ACEi, ARB, Bactrim, Bactrim—marrow suppression.

- Dapsone—Check for G6PD before its use.
- **Cancer**: GI source common—may need EGD / colonoscopy.

Leukopenia: complete workup: *CBC, ANC, peripheral smear, CMV / EBV DNA—PCR, bone marrow biopsy.*

- **Infections**: CMV especially in first six months posttransplant: CMV PCR dx, prophylaxis dependent on risk, can be low with acyclovir or moderate to high, requiring valganciclovir for three to six months. Tx: Ganciclovir IV and granulocyte colony stimulating factor for ANC < $1000/mm^3$.
- **Meds:**
  - ATG, Campath (can cause low counts of CD4+ and CD8+ up to three years).
  - Azathioprine > MMF > CNI—effects on bone marrow suppression.
  - Azathioprine interaction with allopurinol—severe lymphopenia and is contraindicated.
  - Ganciclovir and valganciclovir.
  - Bactrim.
  - MMF and ganciclovir coadministration can lead to reduced nuclear segmentation and excessive clumping of chromatin in neutrophils, aka **Pseudo-Pelger-Huet Anomaly.**

Thrombocytopenia: complete workup: *Plt drop by 50% should be alerting, CBC, peripheral smear, citrated plt, PF4, SRA, DIC panel, hemolytic panel, bone marrow biopsy.*

- **Heparin induced thrombocytopenia (HIT):** 1–3% incidence.
  - Type 1: transient, self-limiting, nonimmunologic.
  - Type 2: IgG / IgM ab to PF4 (plt factor 4 heparin complex) → arterial thrombosis. Presents on day five. Dx: ELISA PF4 (higher sensitivity) or serotonin release

assay (SRA) (higher specificity). Tx: Cessation of heparin and use of direct thrombin inhibitors.

- **Meds:**
  - ATG, mTORi, Azathioprine, MMF.
  - ATGAM worse thrombocytopenia than ATG.
  - Campath.
- **Other:** TTP, ITP, thrombotic microangiopathy, DIC, infections (CMV, Parvovirus B19).

Erythrocytosis: Need to r/o RCC, especially in setting of native cystic kidney disease.

Transplant specific cases:

- **Thrombotic microangiopathy (TMA):** Hemolytic anemia and thrombocytopenia, due to thrombosis of arteriolar and capillary thrombosis. Commonly due to use of CNI (4–15% Cys and 1% tacrolimus), mTORi, AMR, recipient scleroderma, CMV, DCD donors, antiphospholipid syndrome. Tx: PPE, stop CNI, eculizumab used especially in recurrent TMA / complement factor H mutation or antiphospholipid abs.
- Hemophagocytic syndrome (HPS): non–neoplastic macrophages consume RBC / WBC / PLTs due to uncontrolled TNFa and IL-2 stimulation. Dx: five of the eight criteria:
  a. Fever
  b. Cytopenia of at least two lines
  c. Hypertriglyceridemia / Hypofibrinogenemia
  d. Hyperferritinemia
  e. Hemophagocytosis—may need bone marrow biopsy
  f. Elevated IL-2 levels
  g. NK cell decrease
  h. Splenomegaly

  Often associated with infections like EBV / mycobacteria or malignancy.

Treatment: supportive, treat infection, minimize immunosuppression, IVIG, PPE, pulse steroids, sometimes needs transplant nephrectomy.

- **Posttransplantation lymphoproliferative disorder (PTLD):**
  - Has bimodal distribution (early, often immediately posttransplant) and then a second peak four to five years posttransplant.
  - Polyclonal with predominant (85%) B-cell proliferation (less T-cell and NK-cell proliferations) that can lay from a spectrum of hyperplasia to lymphoma.
  - Incidence is 0.5%–1.5%, higher in peds due to higher EBV naive status.
  - Forty percent have BCL6 mutation.
  - Organ transplants have different rates (highest risk is for small intestine transplants, lowest in kidney transplant).
  - Recipient EBV seronegativity is a major risk factor for both early and late PTLD, whereas CMV seronegativity was also associated with early PTLD (CMV synergistic role to EBV).
  - Early PTLD: often related to EBV infection, can be extranodal, and often localized to the transplanted organ (10% of cases). Often is monomorphic lineage, B cell.
  - Late PTLD: often not EBV related, often extranodal. Although it is predominantly B cell, it has a higher percentage T cell.
  - Need to monitor, especially EBV seronegative recipients. Present with fever, night sweats, weight loss, and anorexia, pancytopenia, transaminitis, neurological symptoms.
  - Dx: needs tissue biopsy.
  - Tx:
    - Reduce immunosuppression (decrease CNI trough by 25–50%, stop MMF, can continue with steroids). Takes two to four weeks for response. If no response,

often indicator that it is a poor prognosis. Consider mTORi for immunosuppression instead of CNI.

- Consider antiviral therapy with acyclovir or ganciclovir.
- Rituximab, especially in CD20+ PTLD, started if after six weeks no improvement (three-year survival > 70%). Does not cross BBB, therefore not useful in CNS cases. Will cause a decrease in tumor burden.
- Chemotherapy:
  - CHOP: cyclophosphamide, doxorubicin, vincristine, and prednisone.
  - Intrathecal methotrexate for CNS cases.
- Experimental:
  - Arginine Butyrate: increases EBV / CMV cellular expression and helps antivirals activity.
  - EBV vaccines.

Obesity in Kidney Transplant

BMI ≥ 30 kg/m² obese (40% of the United States), 20% morbidly obese BMI ≥ 35 kg/m².

There is no fudge factor for race (some races distribute the weight differently).
There is an adjustment for amputation.

BMI is not good reflection because:

- AA: More muscle mass than Caucasian.
- Adipose distribution: Central is associated with morbidity.

Thirty-five percent rate of obesity in ESRD.

Effects of obesity:

- Limits dialysis access and associated SSI.
- PD associated with high caloric dialysate and infection rate.

No national BMI limit to transplant (cutoffs are center specific) As UNOS mandates patient and graft survival at one to three years and complications rate, transplanting obese patients can affect a program outcome.

Surgical factors in transplant:

- Obesity—larger incision for exposure, retractor → fat necrosis / longer instruments / head lamps, etc. Longer graft vessels to reach.
- Iliac lymphatics are enlarged with higher risk of lymphocele.

- Longer operative time, higher venous thrombosis—venous compression also procoagulant inflammatory condition.
- Larger superficial and deep SSI (15–44%). Worse five-year patient and graft survival in presence of SSI by 10–15%.
- Pretransplant BMI was an independent predictor of DGF; although DGF is not associated with one year graft survival, it is associated with longer hospital stay, increased health costs, increased radiologic and pathological monitoring and the risk of complications.
- Obese and morbidly obese had higher acute rejection which may be related to difficulty in reaching adequate immunosuppression.
- Seventy-six percent versus 95% one-year graft survival in BMI > 25%.
- There are reports on the effect of BMI on long-term graft survival; where there is often a lower three-year graft survival in obese patients, that is often not significant statistically due to low power.
- Yamamoto et al.: transplanted one kidney in nonobese versus obese. Avg creat was 1.4 versus 2.0 respectively.
- Meier-Kriesche et al.: showed that underweight and morbidly obese had increased risk of death with a functioning graft, although in further analysis this was not true when adjusted for comorbidities.
- Obesity has high leptin secretion by adipocytes →
  - ↑TGF-β → collagen deposition and mesangial proliferation.
  - ↑TNF → glomerulosclerosis.
  - Hyperfiltration injury and proteinuria.
  - ↑Angiotensin II and ↑plasminogen activator inhibitor 1 → endothelial injury and arteriosclerosis.
- Polyoma (BK virus) and rejection is reported more commonly in obese.

- MICS (malnutrition-inflammation complex syndrome): Protein malnutrition secondary to chronic inflammation anorexia and sarcopenia.
- Metabolic syndrome and metabolic transplant DM.

Interventions:

- Diet: 5% of patients were successful with dieting. RF: Food deserts in low S/E groups.
- Exercise: Sedentarism, fatigue/ dyspnea secondary to anemia and hyperlactatemia.
- Bariatric surgery: malabsorption or restriction or both (best results).
  - Diwan et al.: reported in improved candidacy for transplantation but also similar postop outcomes similar to control group in DGF rates, NODAT, readmissions, HTN one-year patient and graft survival.
- Panniculectomy: can be complicated with wound infection.

The obesity paradox:

- BMI did not differentiate between muscle weight versus fat.
- Posttransplant weight loss leads to increased risk of death.
- Assumed BMI drop was related to sarcopenia and deconditioning.
- Wound infection was higher in patients who tried to lose weight immediately before transplant versus those who didn't lose weight.

ESRD etiology and risk of recurrence Posttransplant

DM # 1 Cause ESRD:

- Glomerulosclerosis, **mesangial expansion hallmark**, 30% microalbuminuria will occur at fifteen years of DM.
- **Retinopathy** is mirror of the kidneys damage.
- Eighty to one hundred percent DM nephropathy will recur posttransplant as early as six years—need good glycemic control.
- SPK therefore do better.

HTN:

- Nephrosclerosis is accelerated compared to aging with HTN, especially in AA and when associated with DM.
- RF recurrence posttransplant:
    - DGF, ECD, RAS, native kidneys, CNI, obesity.

GN: UPC monitoring is important.

- **Poststreptococcal:** hallmark hypercellular glomeruli—does not recur.
- **Membranous:** 10–40% recurrence. Subepithelial immune deposits in GBM. Tx: case reports use of rituximab, high dose steroids, and intravenous cyclosporine. ACEi / ARB used to manage proteinuria.
- **MPGN:** associated with Hep C, type I, II, III; 20–50% recurrence but 50–100% in type II (also known as dense deposit disease (DDD). Risk of second recurrence increases to 80% if it has already recurred in first transplant; 15% will lose graft in ten years (two-thirds will lose that in the first two years). Tx: High dose steroids, cyclophosphamide, PPE, and rituximab. Eculizumab

reports of success with DDD type by prevention of membrane attack complex formation.

- **Cryoglobulinemia:** Hep C—often also have hematuria.
- **Primary FSGS:** 20–50% recurrence at first transplant, 100% at second transplant. UPC monitoring necessary. Can recur within first week (suggest a circulating serum factor [suPAR] that injures podocytes). Treatment: plasmapheresis until clinical remission, rituximab, high-dose steroids, and intravenous cyclosporine, oral galactose. Pretransplant plasmapheresis has mixed results but has been shown in pediatric population with lower recurrence.
- **IG-A:** IF large mesangial deposits, aka HSP (if skin, joints, and gut involved); 20–60% recurrence, but doesn't necessary cause ESRD at recurrence. It is believed that 5% of the population has asymptomatic Ig A nephropathy. Tx: ACEi or ARB to decrease proteinuria, high-dose steroids, and cyclophosphamide, (tonsillectomy in a Japanese study). The detrimental effect of recurrent disease is apparent in long-term outcome > ten-year graft survival.
- **HUS/TTP:** 60% recurrence.

Reflux disease: correlates with severity of reflux.

- MC type vesicoureteral reflux:
  - Primary incompetent UVJ.
  - Secondary high pressure in bladder affecting UVJ (e.g., spina bifida).

Autoimmune:

- **Lupus:** MC
  - Recurrence risk quoted at up to 10% at a mean of five years.
  - ANA, dsDNA (needs to be in remission at time of transplant or else high recurrence).
  - Serositis / Raynaud, photosensitivity rash, miscarriage (test coagulation, lupus anticoagulant, and anticardiolipin), alopecia.
  - Diffuse proliferative lupus nephritis (type IV) worst outcome.

- Can recur as early as a week or as late as sixteen years, most within ten years.
- RF AA / Hispanic / Female / Age < thirty-three years.

- **ANCA Vasculitis:**
  - Up to 20% will progress to ESRD despite improved treatment.
  - Recurrence quoted at 10–20% in three years. (Not related to titers of ANCA, type of ANCA, and duration of disease).
  - Wegner versus microscopic polyangiitis, hematuria, crescents present.
  - Even with recurrence is often low severity to lead to graft loss.
- **Anti-glomerular basement membrane disease:**
  - Has a 50% risk of recurrence if positive titers at time of transplant.
  - Best to transplant when patient is in remission for six to twelve months.
  - De-novo anti-GBM can occur in patients with Alport's syndrome and are difficult to treat using conventional treatment and often associated with high recurrence and early recurrence.
- **Atypical hemolytic uremic syndrome and thrombotic microangiopathy (TMA):**
  - Ten percent of HUS is classified as typical as it was not caused by bacterial infection (EHEC) or shiga-like toxins. It is also different from TTP in that it is associated with a normal ADAMTS13 unlike TTP (has < 5% ADAMTS13). TTP also will not show renal biopsy changes while A-HUS will have TMA on kidney biopsy.
  - Dysregulated complement regulatory proteins (e.g., factor H, I, B, C3, and thrombomodulin). Some have anti–factor H ab. Some may be genetically related complement mutation.
  - Fifty percent recurrence as early as first week of transplant. Potentially associated with 80–90% graft loss.

- Tx: PPE, Eculizumab.
- TMA: De novo incidence is 1–10%, can be due to CNI / mTORi, rejection related, and rarely infections like CMV.
- Tx: treatment of cause.

Inherited cystic kidney disease:

- **PCKD:** 80% PKD1 Ch 16, 15% PKD2 Ch 4.
- ADPKD progression RFs genetic, HTN, male, left ventricular mass index, dipstick proteinuria, early onset proteinuria / hematuria. Does not recur posttransplant.
- **Medullary sponge kidney disease:** (good prognosis with normal UPC, but have high stone obstruction risk).
- **Medullary cystic kidney:** (two mutations, type 1 Ch 1, proteinuria, type 2 Ch 16, gout and hyperuricemia. Does not recur.
- **VHL:** (Risk RCC—clear cell type),
- **Tuberous sclerosis** (Vogt triad: seizures / mental retardation / facial angiofibroma—RF for angiomyolipomas and lymphangiomas.

Metabolic disease:

- **Oxalosis: primary:** Hepatic enzyme deficiency, type 1 MC, alanine: glyoxylate aminotransferase deficiency. Type 2: glycoxylate reductase deficiency. Difficult to prevent recurrence, best when combined with liver transplant. **Secondary:** malabsorption, chronic pancreatitis. Lowering oxalate in diet and pancreatic enzyme replacement.
- **Fabry's disease:** deficiency of α-galactosidase A. Metabolic deposit and damage eyes, autonomic nervous system, CVS, and kidneys. No recurrence with enzyme replacement therapy.

Transplant Nephrectomy:

Early: Hyperacute thrombosis, early acute rejection, severe infection—leave a cuff of donor artery and vein. Extracapsular resection, keep foley, and JP drain.

Late: 79% require it.

- Benefits:
  - Reversal of chronic inflammation, lower CRP, higher albumin, decrease EPO requirement (graft could result in EPO resistance). Stopping immunosuppression → reduce infection / CVD / malignancy / clearance of BK virus. Relieve recurrent pain.
- Risks: Bleeding, healing, allosensitization.
- Approach:
  - Intracapsular approach and clamp hilum—oversew with 4.0 Prolene. Remove bladder urothelium to allow cure for BKV.
  - Stop CNI and rapid steroid taper.
  - Always check for femoral pulse.
  - Prefer to close with nonabsorbable sutures.

Reproduction and Transplant

ESRD: results often in anovulation in women in the reproductive age group, also leads to early menopause. Men have defective gonadal function and are also infertile.

Transplantation: will often reverse the above process.

Meds and reproduction:

Sirolimus can lead to male infertility and should be avoided in men interested in having children.

Valganciclovir is teratogenic.

Mycophenolate mofetil and mycophenolic acid associated with structural development changes.

Contraception counseling: in the peritransplant period is very important in women. In men, however, the gonadal system does not appear to be affected with germ cell mutations from immunosuppressive meds.

Previously IUD were contraindicated in transplant recipients due to pelvic inflammatory risk, but newer IUD don't have this increased risk.

Two barrier method recommended versus combination of hormonal and barrier methods or irreversible contraception with tubal ligation or male vasectomy.

Pregnancy:

Per American Society of Transplantation, it should be delayed after one year of transplant.

It can be considered within the first year only if:

- Stable graft function

- No rejection
- Good allograft function (creat < 1.5 and proteinuria < 500 mg/day).
- Not on teratogenic meds
- No history of active CMV infections

Risks during pregnancy:
Accelerated graft dysfunction: correlated with graft function at time of conception, so not at increased risk if graft function was good (defined as **creat < 1.5 and proteinuria < 500 mg/day**).
Rejection rates in pregnant versus nonpregnant are the same and are treated the same way—methylpred (ATG and Simulect use has been reported).

Need to continue with immunosuppressive meds with close monitoring to levels as volume distribution changes in pregnancy.

Renal dysfunction might be hard to pick up early as normally in pregnancy the intravascular volume and GFR increases.

Increased risk of HTN. (Cannot use ACEi or ARB as associated with intrauterine growth retardation IUGR.) Preferred treatment is methyl-dopa.
Preeclampsia in one-third of maternal transplant pregnancies, lower if they never had HTN (5%). Close monitoring is required.

Infant risks:
Preterm birth risk in 50% of cases and at thirty-six weeks mean gestational age.

Low birth weight < 2.5 kg in 50% of cases.

IUGR: defined as being less than tenth percentile for gestational age, often associated with decreased cognitive function in adulthood.

Long-term outcomes are not clear. One study suggests neurocognitive and autoimmune disease increased risks.

Delivery:

Normal vaginal delivery recommended, unless contraindicated from an obstetrical point of view.

Breast feeding:

No clear recommendations for or against it.

Selective Transplant Infections

Generally immunosuppressed patients are at higher vulnerability for infections but also deteriorate faster. Workup of any pathology should take into account the possibility of infectious etiology, as these patients can get atypical presentations (masked by the immunosuppression) but also can involve activation of latent pathogens, develop opportunistic infections, or even have coinfections.

Infectious etiology varies with time, from transplant.

First month postop: technical related, nosocomial related, or latent infection from donor / recipient.
Months two through six: Latent reactivation of infection (relapsed, latent, or opportunistic).
Months > six: Community acquired infections.

Generally decreasing immunosuppression is the first-line therapy that should precede direct antimicrobial therapy.

BK Virus

Virology:

- Polyoma Virus: dsDNA, nonenveloped.
  - SV40: no human disease known-transmitted through polio vaccine.
  - JC virus: associated with PML. Rarely cause a nephropathy similar to BK.
  - WU / KI viruses: Respiratory tract disease.
  - BK: Hemorrhagic cystitis and nephropathy.
    - Initial infection at three to four years of age, 100% by ten years.
    - Initial respiratory- or GI-like infection
    - Disseminates by remaining latent in uroepithelium.
    - Four subtypes based on VP1 gene.

Pathogenesis in renal transplant:

- Ineffective immune surveillance.
- Absence of prior recipient immunity to BK (i.e., recipient [–] donor [+]).
- Molecular variability of T and VP1 proteins.
- Alloimmune activation to HLA mismatch triggers BK nephropathy.

Risk Factors:

HLA mismatch
Previous acute rejection, especially if ATG was used.
Female donor.
Male recipient.
Advanced recipient age.
High tacrolimus levels or prolonged MMF.

Use of ureteral stents periop period.
DM.
SPK higher than kidney alone.
SLK is lower than kidney alone.
Cadaveric donor higher than living donor.
High BMI.

Signs or symptoms:

- Asymptomatic viruria.
- Hemophagocytic syndrome (fever, pancytopenia + elevated LDH, ALT, TG).
- Multiorgan disease in severe reactivations.
- Hemorrhagic cystitis (70% of HSCT). Mild to life threatening, mainly type I BKV.
- Ureteral stenosis (less common) 4%.
- BK nephropathy (interstitial nephritis) and graft loss.
- Autoimmune versus malignancies (bladder cancer).

In many cases asymptomatic viruria is seen one to three months prior to BK nephropathy.
Is seen in 5% of kidney transplants.

Diagnosis usually on screening:

- Urine cytology—decoy cells (not used now).
- DNA detection in urine or blood (popular).
  - Urine 10^7 copies, blood 5–10^3 copies/ml high risk of developing BK nephropathy.
  - Repeat testing is needed.
  - Variance in logs between test centers is important to note, especially if different labs are used.
- SV40 staining on biopsy. Described as pattern:
  - Minimal inflammation
  - B-TCN +/– acute rejection-like.
  - Chronic allograft nephropathy like with moderate to severe fibrosis.

Screening allows to adjust and decrease the level of immunosuppression (IS).

Treatment:

- Decrease IS:
  - Either by decreasing trough level of FK < 6 / MMF < 1 g/day.
  - Discontinuing one drug FK / MMF.
    - Some have reported better responses with MMF reduction in dosing / some groups have advocated switching Prograf to cyclosporine (as this, too, decreases MMF absorption).
  - Switching to mTOR: associated with lower viral infectious risk.
- Cidofovir:
  - Does not affect BK virus directly.
  - Restores p53 and pRB, allowing apoptosis of infected cells.
  - Associated variable responses with decrease in VL but potential nephrotoxicity, cytopenias, and ocular hypotony.
- Leflunomide: has antiviral activity.
  - Associated with lower viral load extracellularly but with variable clinical outcome changes.
  - levels of blood concentration 40 mg/ml but associated with adverse reaction with TMA, hepatotoxicity.
- Fluoroquinolones:
  - Variable response, dose dependent.
  - Aids in decreasing viral load in bladder and proximal tubular epithelium.
  - Prophylactic ciprofloxacin has been shown to decrease incidence of severe hemorrhagic cystitis in HSCT and in some kidney transplant series. Where one-month postop ciprofloxacin was associated with lower three month but not at twelve months.

- Acts to inhibit T ag helicase activity.
- IVIG:
    - Very variable response.
    - Often used if concomitant rejection in addition to steroids or as rescue therapy in those who fail to improve despite IS changes.
- Need for retransplant:
    - If graft is lost.
    - Higher risk of recurrence—quoted at 35% in one study.
    - Recommend that retransplants are done with undetectable or low viremia / viruria.
    - Transplant nephrectomy of failed graft may be considered but is not necessary for successful transplantation.
    - The patients would need higher monitoring / surveillance after transplantation.

CMV Infection

- Eighty to ninety percent of the population infected.
- Primary from donor can cause mono-like syndrome.
- Reactivation of latent infection.
- Super / coinfection
- Affect PMNs and macrophages, fibroblasts, smooth muscle, and endothelial cells.
- Will need to graft vascular vasculopathy and rejection.
- Risk factors:
  - HLA mismatch—allograft stimulation
  - Allograft rejection
  - CMV (R– D+)
  - Depleting induction agents
  - Immunosuppression
- Management:
  - No prophylaxis was associated with > 50% infection risk, reduced to 4% when antiviral prophylaxis was used.
  - Biweekly monitoring is recommended in immediate periop or after rejection treatment.
  - IMPACT trial studying duration of antiviral prophylaxis:
    - High risk (D+/R–) had lower one-year and two-year CMV infections, showed two hundred days versus one hundred days of prophylaxis, had lower one-year and two-year CMV infection risk (21% versus 39%), with similar rejection rates, CMV resistance and other infection rates.
      - Many centers use six months of ganciclovir for this subgroup.

    - Moderate risk group (D+/R+, D–/R+) often are on prophylaxis for three months
    - Low risk group (D–/R–) are covered with acyclovir for one month. Acyclovir inferior CMV effect and better at herpes / shingles prevention.
- Drugs:
  - Valganciclovir: has a better bioavailability (dosed as 900 mg daily—like treatment dose) than ganciclovir, and although the CMV infections rates were the same for both, valganciclovir:
    - Had delayed onset of CMV viremia and infection versus ganciclovir.
    - Had higher neutropenia (8%) versus ganciclovir (3%).
    - Needs to be renally dosed.
    - Antiviral therapy was also associated with a 51% decreased bacterial and 38% fungal infections.
  - CMV IVIG, aka Cytogam:
    - In the preganciclovir era it was used as prophylaxis agents.
    - It is not recommended as a sole agent but can be considered in addition to antiviral use for prophylaxis.
    - It is recommended in high risk transplants of thoracic / intestinal and liver prophylaxis.
    - Role in kidney transplant not very clear but should be considered:
      - Rescue / adjunctive therapy—in leukopenic patients due to mycophenolate or valganciclovir.
      - Or for those under intense immunosuppression (rejection treatments with high-dose steroids or depleting agents).
      - In some trials was used in CMV pneumonitis treatment in addition to antiviral with generally improved outcomes.

  - No consensus on dosing.
- Foscarnet:
  - Reserved for CMV resistance cases.
- Cidofovir:
  - Due to toxicity, left as last resource.
  - Has no direct CMV activity.

Rejection Immunology

Hyperacute:

- Preformed Ab.
- Type II hypersensitivity reaction.
- Occurs minutes to hours posttransplant.
- ABO incompatible transplants.

Accelerated Acute:

- Presensitized T cells to recipient antigen.
- Memory T cells activated.
- Secondary response.
- Occurs within one week of transplant.

Acute rejection:

- Naive B cells or T cells interacting with transplant antigen.
- Primary response.
- Occurs within one week to six months.
- Can be humoral or cellular immune response.

Chronic rejection:

- Delayed response (months to years).
- T cells or B cells active to minor antigen constantly at a low grade.
- Repeated acute injuries.
- Organs damage secondary to vasculopathy and fibrosis.
- Also same mechanism for graft-versus-host disease (GvHD).
    - Graft (donor) T cells / B cells attack recipient antigens.

The ability to predict adequate immunosuppression that can decrease rejection and infection has been a research interest.

There is research studying recipient blood lipid profile as a potential predictor for first year rejection. A study found that patients with ACR/ ABMR in first year did have a similar lipid profile versus patients who did not develop this in the first year of transplant.

The levels of donor-derived cell-free DNA may be used as a precursor for subclinical level of injury / rejection and is used in some centers as adjunct clinically to guide overall monitoring of grafts.

In one trial the torque teno virus (TTN) is a virus that is prevalent in 99% of solid organ transplants. It is a surrogate to both cellular and humoral immunity, and certain low thresholds were associated with increased risk of rejection, and higher thresholds were predictable of infection. This reached a steady state value that can be used three months postop and could be used in the future to monitor and tailor immunosuppression.

Transplant Rejection

Graft injury (necessary regardless of inflammatory cells present or not).

- Acute rejection: fast and efficient response.
  - T-cell mediated
  - Antibody mediated
  - Proinflammatory cytokine mediated
- Chronic: slower and inefficient effector response.
  - T-cell mediated
  - Dysregulated repair mechanism (endothelial repair alteration)
  - Antibody mediated
  - Nonimmune damage
  - Recurrent disease misdiagnosed as chronic rejection

More important to know mechanism of rejection rather than acuteness to help treat it.

- Cellular effector mechanism:
  - T cell release of perforin and granzymes, leading to cytotoxicity.
  - Naive T cells are not active and have a higher threshold to reach in order to activate versus memory T cells that are more primed to activate on APC encounter, have already matured in secondary lymphoid tissue.
  - Heterologous immunity: when a T cell is active due to an antigen, the system is revved up such that other antigens have a higher chance of eliciting a large response—the system is revved up even though it might not be the initial antigen. This increases the chance that a T cell will develop cross-reaction to other antigens.

    - This population of naive (hard-to-activate) and memory (easy-to-activate) changes with age as neonates have more of the naive form versus adults have more of the memory form and so transplanting in those age groups has a different immunological process.
- Acellular Effector Mechanisms:
    - Hyper acute rejection: Preexisting host antibodies to antigens, leading to inflammation and vascular thrombosis.
    - Alloantibody reaction variables:
        - Isotype of antibody IgG1 / IgM best at complement fixation.
        - Titer level.
        - Target cell adaption: hard if massive acute response versus chronic antibody response.
        - Antigen distribution: Organ usually express MHC-1, but in reperfusion of organs, MHC-II is upregulated and expressed.
    - Complement:
        - C3 / C5-MAC is a critical target for drugs.
    - Cytokines and complement activation can lead to rejection phenotype even in the absence of T cells.
    - In fact, cell infiltration is not sufficient to reflect rejection. Type of cells is more important; macrophages are a worse marker of injury than lymphocytes.
    - This is why we see tubulitis as a marker of rejection on biopsy—the tubules epithelium cytokine release leads to chemotaxis and tubules infiltration with T cells.
    - T cells the cytokines release may still give a rejection phenotype with absent T cells.
    - Platelets are important source CD154, and therefore affect immune response, which is why reperfusion and innate graft injury can dramatically affect the allogenic response.

Transplant Rejection Biopsy Changes

Range of biopsy findings:

1. Normal
2. Hyperacute rejection
3. Borderline changes
4. Acute rejection
    a. Grade 1 = mild, Grade 2 = moderate with (A/B = intimal arteritis presence).
    b. Grade 3 = Severe arteritis, transmural arteritis with fibrinoid change, focal infarction / hemorrhage.
5. Chronic allograft nephropathy:
    a. Grade 1–3 = mild to severe, interstitial fibrosis / tubular atrophy (IFTA)
6. Other:
    a. Toxicity, infection, ATN, disease recurrence, etc.

Scoring each of the features below from zero to three depending on severity, leads to the rejection grading:

- T = tubulitis
- I = inflammation
- V = intimal arteritis
- G = glomerulitis

Tubulitis and vasculitis are the principal indication of acute cellular rejection not inflammation.

Score is based on seeing the worst tubule under H/E—number of lymphocytes per tubule.

Lesion	0	1	2	3
t	None	1-4 cells/cross section	5-10 cells/ cross section	>10 cells/ cross section
i	None	Up to 25%	Up to 50%	>50% of parenchyma
v	None	Mild-moderate	Moderate-severe	Severe, with transmural changes, fibrinoid necrosis

Acute Cellular Rejection:

- IA/B—based on t2–3—tubulitis with no arteritis.
- II A/B—based on V1–2—mild to moderate arteritis even if no tubulitis.
- III—V3—Severe or transmural arteritis.

Acute Antibody Mediated Rejection:

- Three criteria:
  - Morphologic acute tissue injury:
    - ATN injury
    - Neutrophil / mononuclear—peritubular capillaries / glomeruli / capillary thrombosis / TMA
    - Arteritis
  - Immunopathologic evidence of antibody action:
    - C4d deposition:
      - Immunohistochemical is less sensitive than immunofluorescence.
      - Importance is not validated as AMR can fix complement without C4d deposition.
  - Serologic evidence—DSA/ antidonor endothelial antigen spike

Chronic Allograft Nephropathy:

- Severity based on interstitial fibrosis (ci) and tubular atrophy (ct).

- Grade 1 / II / III—mild / moderate/ severe.
- These changes may be associated with features of antibody mediated or cellular mediated rejections, making them chronic active antibody rejection or chronic active T-cell mediated rejection, respectively.

Grade	Histology	Interstitial Fibrosis	Tubular Atrophy
I	mild	ci1 6-25% cortex	ct1 25% of cortex
II	moderate	ci2 26-50% cortex	ct2 26-50% of cortex
III	severe	ci3 >50%	ct3 >50% of cortex

Other:

Diabetic nodular glomerulosclerosis: in donor biopsy is a contraindication to use, milder diabetic changes can be used.
CNI toxicity: newly developing nodular arteriolar hyalinosis and stripped fibrosis.
BKV: SV40 stain.
CMV: eosinophilic inclusions "owl's eye" appearance.
FSGS: can recur within hours of transplantations, associated with rising proteinuria.
Acute pyelonephritis: purulent casts, many neutrophil cells.
Fungal infections: mononuclear cells mainly and stains.
Thrombotic microangiopathy (TMA): in acute setting can be related to:

- AMR
- CNI toxicity
- HUS
- Ischemic injury

Transplant Rejection Treatment

Immediate graft rejection due to preformed donor specific antibodies:

- ABO antibodies
- Donor-specific anti-HLA
- Xenoreactive ab

Initiates as early as intraoperative and is complete within hours to days.
B cells activated undergo clonal expansion and produce Ig that bind the antigen and endothelium, resulting in complement activation and inflammation and thrombosis.

Prevention:

- Historically is by appropriate crossmatching
- Currently is by reducing pretransplant antibody titers and posttransplant titers.

Antibody-reducing therapies:

- Plasmapheresis:
  - Loss of molecular weight-based extracorporeal hemofiltration, which includes also clotting factors as well as Ig.
- Immunadsorption:
  - Biologic activity–based hemofiltration columns that bind to *specific ab* (*very selective*).
  - Staphylococcal Protein A—binding HLA ab or even ABO ab.
- IVIG:

    - Polyclonal IgG from healthy blood donor serum (as much as five thousand).
    - Immunomodulators by antagonizing and neutralizing anti-HLA activity.
    - Modulates complement activity.
    - Inhibits B and T call function.
    - Response is variable—weaker in patients with high titers, some are even nonresponders.

B-cell ablation therapies:

- Splenectomy:
    - Debulk plasma cell (activated B cell) reservoir.
    - However, spleen is not only reservoir.
    - Mainly currently used as a rescue strategy in combination with antibody removal strategy.
- Rituximab:
    - Anti-CD20 on B cells not seen on plasma cells, which are the active form.
    - Not a monotherapy.
- Bortezomib:
    - Anti-NFKB: toxic to plasma cells. Helps reduce DSA and plasma cells. FDA approved for multiple myeloma-used as an off-label drug.
- Eculizumab:
    - Monoclonal ab Anti-C5: prevents MAC formation by complement and is used to prevent end-organ injury.
    - Highest potential in hyperacute rejection.
- Auxiliary partial liver transplant:
    - Acts like a sponge absorbing the DSA ab and protecting other transplanted organs.
- Hyperacute rejection is rarely seen in liver

Treatment of ACR:

Type 1A/B = often require pulsed steroid (500 mg methylprednisolone, three doses) therapy and increasing immunosuppression.

Type 2 and above will, in addition, require depleting agent, also, most commonly using Thymoglobulin. These patients are at increased risk of infections and will need a fine balance of sufficient IS without increased risk of infections.

Treatment of AMR:
Clinical AMR treatment:

Eighty to ninety percent reversal associated with use of plasmapheresis +/– IVIG, (Tacrolimus + MMF) based maintenance.
Rituximab +/– above regimen was associated with high success rate but also associated with higher infectious risk, especially JC progressive multifocal leukoencephalopathy.
Campath / Bortezomib / Eculizumab: have all been studied with AMR treatment (see desensitization chapter).
Some features of cellular rejection may be present, requiring pulsed steroids or even depleting agents.

Subclinical AMR treatment:

Although controversial, more studies are in support of treating subclinical AMR. Although the type of treatment is unclear, most have given a form pulsed steroids and increase in baseline immunosuppression.
Twenty-five percent of low-risk patients will develop de novo DSA.
Studies have shown that de novo DSA has been a strong predictor of rejection. In one study, 53% of patients with normal graft function who developed de novo DSA had rejection changes on biopsy.
Rush et al. untreated subclinical rejection was associated with early chronic pathology and late graft dysfunction.
Presence of DSA is associated with a nine-fold higher increased risk of rejection than those without DSA.
Among previously unsensitized patients, de novo DSA against HLA class II predominates in renal transplant recipients.

Donor HLA-DR mismatch and nonadherence to immunosuppressive medications have been shown to be strong predictors of de novo DSA.

Some have found that treated subclinical AMR has similar graft survival compared to those without AMR, but untreated subclinical AMR was associated with higher rates of graft loss.

Standardized DSA monitoring is essential.

DSA MFI cutoff values are variable to type of DSA but should always be considered as part of the clinical picture, as some low level DSA maybe.

Low threshold for biopsying kidneys with de novo DSA even with normal graft function.

Index

CPSIA information can be obtained
at www.ICGtesting.com
Printed in the USA
BVHW041139041220
594901BV00020B/444

9 781649 905956